Health and Medicine
in the Lutheran Tradition

Health/Medicine and the Faith Traditions

Edited by Martin E. Marty and Kenneth L.Vaux

Health/Medicine and the Faith Traditions
explores the ways in which major religions
relate to the questions of human well-being.
It issues from Project Ten,
an international program of the
Lutheran General Medical Center
in Park Ridge, Illinois.

Health and Medicine in the Lutheran Tradition

BEING WELL

Martin E. Marty

CROSSROAD · NEW YORK

1986

The Crossroad Publishing Company
370 Lexington Avenue, New York, N.Y. 10017

Library of Congress Cataloging in Publication Data

Marty, Martin E., 1928–
Health and medicine in the Lutheran tradition.
1. Health—Religious aspects—Lutheran Church.
2. Medicine—Religious aspects—Lutheran Church.
3. Lutheran Church—Doctrines.   I. Title.
BX8074.H42M37 1983   261.5′6   83–15231
ISBN 0-8245-0613-8

To Ursula
daughter
on the highest step

Contents

Preface

This book, which we believe to be the first on its subject in the over 450 years of Lutheran history, would not exist were it not for the company of concerns among numbers of faiths. Thanks to the impetus of my colleague Kenneth Vaux, Lutheran General Hospital, through its Human Values Forum, has used its Park Ridge, Illinois, base to establish what was code-named "Project Ten" or "Project X." That "X" was to stand for "ten," since we were to explore the way ten faith traditions handled ten generic themes related to well-being. By now the X means X, the unknown, since more faiths and more themes have come into view, and since we are coming to know better that we do not yet know much about how faith traditions and well-being connect.

Project X seeks to "assemble, assess, and apply the wisdom of the faith traditions, the medical community, and other caring professions to issues of health care faced by individuals, families and society." We are working through three phases. Underway is a very elaborate set of historical essays on these traditions. As a historian on the project, I find the subject of these essays in my area of purview. Yet this book, along with a number of similar volumes on other faith traditions, moves beyond the "data-base" approach of the historical essays and beyond "assembling," to "assessing." The books in this series seek to connect past with present, far with near, farfetched with urgently close and appropriate. What is the current state of the traditions? Have they anything to say to the issue of well-being?

Within the limits of space dictated by the series format, one is confined and must leave out some important elements. Thus I have chosen not to go into great detail on certain aspects of technical "bioethics," in which Lutheran insights might be applied to homosexuality, genetic experimenting, or organ transplants. The literature on medical ethics is vast and rapidly expanding. Instead I chose to accent the *theological understandings that are antecedent to moral discourse and ethical choice and to elements of behavior and care*, which are often not the subject of professionals in medical ethics.

The first phase of the project is designed chiefly for professional people in the worlds of medicine and religion. This second phase, while seeking to include them also, moves forthrightly into a second zone. We are seeking to reach the lay people, lay in respect both to the clergy in religion and to the medical experts in the realm of physical well-being. We hope that they will use the books to compare their lives with their tradition—or, when they read outside their own traditions, to learn from what others might carry to them.

As I wrote, I had in mind as readers of these books informed lay people, pastors, nurses, deaconesses, teachers, and physicians. Wherever possible, authors in this phase of the project are to avoid technical terminology and to keep the sometimes forbidding kinds of scholarly apparatus to a minimum. I have tried to acknowledge my major borrowings in the footnotes without providing documentation in wearying detail in order to impress those who are impressed by mere volume of footnotes.

A third phase of the project, which as I write remains "projected" since it is necessarily expensive in a time when funds for humane programs are hard to come by, would "apply" the lore and learning in the clinical situation. Lutheran General Hospital, a pioneer agency in this field because of its Human Ecology base concept, is intended to be the theater of operations for this phase. Periodically, teams of professionals in medicine, religion, ethics, and care will, it is hoped, be enabled to converge on the hospital for sustained periods of time. They are to be chartered to interact with each other, with the staff, and within the boundaries of the appropriate, with patients. Out of it may come an almost encyclopedic approach to this subject.

Those who would like to read more about the assumptions of the project will find a collection of essays in Martin E. Marty and Kenneth L. Vaux, *Health/Medicine and the Faith Traditions* (Philadelphia: Fortress, 1982). Since Vaux and I wrote less than 100 of the 350 pages, we can point with pride to work by others and concur that readers of our books in the present series will also get much from what these others have written in our jointly edited book. It is a pioneering effort, which sets forth assumptions, preliminary findings, and helpful clues about well-being.

Since volumes like this one are to connect clinic and academy with congregation, I am happy to acknowledge the many kinds of support given the project by the congregation of Grace Lutheran Church, River Forest, Illinois. Its pastor, Dr. F. Dean Lueking, has been a participant from the beginning. Through his efforts and through the generosity of Mrs. Bernice Feicht, a parishioner, funds were made available to carry through to completion the planning, research, writing, and publication of this series opener.

Through the propinquity of the Vaux and Marty homes, the friendship of our families, and the commonness of our interests, Vaux was able to draw me into this field, which was native to him and remote to me. As a mid-career historian of religion, however, I found it appropriate as an area of study. Today people in my profession are moving from an old set of curiosities to new ones. Once upon a time "church history" meant histories of bishops and monks, theologians and parsons, constitutions and prayer book revisions. Today, thanks to the women's revolution, the new techniques of social history, and myriad other impetuses, we are learning to write "people's history."

Such history is more intimate, closer to home and congregation. It involves histories of families and ethnic clusters, of attitudes toward sexuality and the stages of life, and, as evidenced here, of care and the search for well-being. This book has permitted me to fuse my pastoral and personal interests with my professional and professorial inquiries.

Crucial to the project are the researches of two colleagues. Mary-Carroll Sullivan, "research consultant," is assembling literally hundreds of thousands of book and article titles on the Lutheran General computers, a data bank supreme. This has made her a kind of walking expert on the subject, and she has been always ready with help. Similarly, my research assistant at The University of Chicago, R. Scott Appleby, has interrupted his own dissertation writing and college teaching to do research helpful for these pages. I thank them both, as well as my wife, Harriet, who made many valuable editorial suggestions.

Pastors Lawrence E. Holst and David T. Stein serve as project chairman and project administrator under Mr. George Caldwell, president of Lutheran General Hospital. Without their vision Project Ten would never have been launched and without their zeal it would not have reached Phase Two. Let them represent the several members of the team who have been of help. They will be much called upon in the future as the project develops. They join me in commending to you this sampling of the many deep, rich, fluid, and problematic faith traditions, and in hoping that it may contribute to human well-being.

MARTIN E. MARTY
The University of Chicago
Theological Consultant to Project Ten

"I have nothing but praise for the physicians who adhere closely to their principles. But they should not take it amiss if I cannot always agree with them, for they wish to make a fixed star out of me when I am a roving planet. The responsibility of physicians, to whom human life is entrusted, is a great one. Since our bodies contain many mysterious vapors and internal and invisible organs, there are also various and unexpected dangers; our bodies can go to pieces in an hour. Therefore, a physician must be humble. . . ."

—Martin Luther, 1538

"We must . . . regard the sacrament . . . as a pure, wholesome, soothing medicine which aids and quickens us in both soul and body. For where the soul is healed, the body has benefited also."

—Martin Luther,
Large Catechism

Part I

WELLNESS AND ILLNESS

·1·

Traditions and
the Lutheran Tradition

FAITH TRADITIONS AND "BEING WELL"

"Are you saved?"

"How are you?"

People in the Lutheran tradition traditionally do not ask the first of these two questions. They do, however, *think* it about themselves and those they love. Not all faiths are, like theirs, a religion of salvation. Buddhism and Hinduism, for example, have different gifts to offer. Christianity does focus on saving people. No branch of this faith is more concerned than the Lutheran with making the claim that it would help believers be "right with God." Evangelical Lutherans consider the supreme question of life to be the relation of people to their Maker. They believe that human beings only have well-being if God takes action to save them from whatever ill they fall heir to or evil they commit.

"Are you saved?"

"How are you?"

People with Lutheran habits habitually *do* ask the second question. Of course, they would not have to be religious, Christian, or of Lutheran heritage to do so. A natural human instinct leads us to greet others with at least casual concern about their health and well-being. "How are you?" usually means "Are you well?" Most mortals consider being well the second most important question of life. They do not ordinarily ask, "Are you wealthy?" At street corner meetings few would begin a chat with a query about the social status of another person. Friends want to know whether those they meet have a sense of bodily health and feel at home with the world around them. "Yes, I am quite well, thank you!" is the response of someone who looks out on a good day and is not worried about tomorrow.

"I'm well, thank you!"

"I'm saved!"

When answers to the two questions come, we should rank them in this reverse order. So say cynics. They would disagree with the proposal that

3

being well is only the *second* most urgent element in life. If you have your health, you can have many other things, argue the critics of faith. You can even have the luxury of being religious!

Persons can test their health. Are the bodily parts functioning well? Is there an absence of pain? Is there suffering? Is there a positive sense of "being at home" in the world? If you can answer yes to all these questions, everything else follows. You should have the ability to earn enough to put a roof over your head, clothes on your back, and food in your stomach. The suspicious questioner of faith will not believe that anyone honestly ranks anything higher than such well-being. A member of the medical profession, who usually sees people during times of disease, is likely to share the suspicions. Pain and fear have ways of blocking out secondary interests.

"I'm saved."

"I'm well, thank you!"

Christian believers, among them Lutherans, insist that this is the right sequence of concerns. Of course, they would say, an agnostic or an unbeliever can enjoy bodily health and feel good. Those, however, who believe that God in Christ gives eternal life and in love has removed the barriers between the divine and the human rank "being saved" ahead of "being well."

This ranking can also be tested. Believers all recognize that the only thing they know for sure about their future is that they will die. That thought should disturb their sense of well-being. If they are "saved," however, they are free to be less concerned about the disturbance. People of faith know that terrible suffering and pain are likely someday to come their way. Of course, they hope to be spared these evils. Yet their prayer in the long night watches is that God will save them in the midst of suffering. They plead that their Maker will not be distant in their hour of need. Nothing shall separate them from the love of God in Christ. Concern for being well can then occupy their minds.

"*How* are you saved?"

"*How* do you stay well?"

Not all people ask the first of these questions. "Being saved" is a goal on which Christians agree. *How* one is saved is the issue that inspires argument among them. Believers often disagree about the various means of coming to be right with God. Lutherans like to think that no other group of Christians is more eager than they to say that being saved is a free gift of God, to which humans in turn make a response. Sometimes they accuse others unjustly and sometimes they point out justly that other Christians stress chiefly the human part of salvation. In such cases persons are saved through their own efforts to do good. At this moment, the point is simply that different heritages of faith have different ways of answering questions about being saved.

"How do you stay well?" is a question that people quite readily ask each other. They may be timid about issues of faith. Most are unready to argue about them. They are fearless and ready to go, however, with comments about being well. Casual strangers who meet waste only a few seconds before they compare diets and health regimens. "Let me tell you about my operation." That opening sentence dooms many an acquaintance to a drearily detailed story about how the partner in conversation came back from ill health. Friends compare notes about how many miles they jog, how many teeth they have filled, which therapy regimen suits their nerves, or how to insure the best medical care. Physicians can report on how seriously patients take medical counsel.

Answers to questions about how people are saved depend in part on the traditions to which they belong. In the modern world these traditions increasingly overlap. They feed into each other. They blend. Even to this day, nevertheless, the textbooks on how Catholics are saved differ from those of Methodism, Lutheranism, or Seventh-Day Adventism. Generations of leaders and teachers find special ways of talking about how to be right with God. Parents bring up children using the inherited language that comes along with these ways. Elders instill in their young some habits that go along with this language. Particular songs and hymns express these ways.

Sometimes rules and regulations go along with the issue of salvation. If you want to be saved, then do not eat this food on that day. Go to church, confess your sins, receive the sacrament, be good, feel free. Doctors and nurses have to learn if some of these rules apply to their patients in matters of healing.

People today are free to believe whatever they wish about religious words, habits, and rules. Yet if they belong to families of faith, they tend to respond to them in partly predictable and patterned ways. Believers in their practices have something in common with others of the same tradition.

As for the believers' second most urgent question, how they are to be well, some answers may also come in package deals. More than many realize, most people seek well-being as members of communities, as heirs of traditions. Their sense of tradition begins on the most intimate level, in the family. Some families curse their own children with ill-being because the parents are child abusers or sexual molesters. Scientists and researchers are discovering that these evils often "run in the family." Child abusers were often themselves abused when they were children. People can break the chain between generations, but they have to know that they are links in such a chain. Some medical analysts say that the disease of alcoholism also can "run in the family." Alcoholic parents sometimes seem to lead or drive their children to drink. Medical personnel and counselors try to help disrupt this passing on of a habit through generations.

Disease can come in traditions. Only parents in dark-skinned races pass sickle-cell anemia on to their children. Some diseases afflict people of Jewish heritage. Members of certain inbred rural sects such as the Amish have too small a pool of potential spouses on which to draw. They may pass on to their young genetically derived problems. A medical researcher can see in this way of transmitting health problems something that compares to the way Christians see all members of the human race passing on the evil that is in them—the tendency to sin.

Being ill and being well are not only parts of genetic tendencies within a blood tradition. There are other conscious ways in which the family hands down good health or ill health. Some households are prone to hypochondria. Parents teach their children to be obsessed with illness. These children pass their hypochondria on to later generations. Other families have a tradition of good health. They take pains to exercise and provide for leisure and vacations. They create a climate in which people do not have to inflict ill-being on each other through the use of hateful words. The family can be a group way of defining being well.

So is the tribe or the nation. If a medical missionary tries to cure someone with whose ways she is not familiar, someone expert in those ways may say, "No, that is not *done* among this people." Some tribal people consult what outsiders call the witch doctor or the medicine man. What they do comes to be written about as "traditional medicine." When Christian physicians come to what is for them a new tribe or nation, they soon learn that they are confronting traditions of care. Healers from the Western world have to learn about herbs, potions, spells, and seasons before they can bring some kind of modern hospital care.

What the helpful intruders often overlook or forget is that to the people they would serve these newcomers, these Christians, also represent a tradition. In the Western Christian tradition healers are likely to blend ancient prayer and modern medicine. They welcome tools of science and instruments of faith. Not all the world does this. For that matter, not even all Christian traditions do so.

On Western soil it is easiest to say that a question such as "*How* are you well?" can be answered best in traditions of faith where health is itself the subject of extensive teachings. You may not have detailed knowledge of Christian Science. However, anyone who knows anything at all about it knows that Christian Scientists have a special tradition through which they see the issue of being saved along with being well. Seventh-Day Adventism, which promotes vegetarianism, has a very distinct health lore within Christianity. Jehovah's Witnesses are well known for seeing salvation and well-being tied to a system that does not allow for blood transfusions. Students of health patterns find fewer instances of cancer and more instances of longer life among Latter-Day Saints or Mormons than among the "Gentiles" who surround them. Analysts account for this tendency by saying that the Mormon tradition has certain teachings and practices that promote health—such as refraining from alcohol, smoking, or even the use of caffeine.

Observant Jews may seek salvation and well-being along lines of traditions that go all the way back to the Hebrew Scriptures, which were written more than two thousand years ago. Within mainstream Christianity, Roman Catholicism has traditions of health and well-being that are reflected in special views of sexuality and the care of life.

The closer one comes to home, the more difficult it is to recognize a tradition. There is an old story about a man who is surprised to find out that he always spoke in prose. And then there are those about men and women who come to find that what they thought the whole human race did, or what all Christians practiced, belonged only to their own much smaller part of the tradition. People in tribes that others used to call primitive or traditional do not think of themselves as primitive. They do not necessarily even know of other traditions. They do not see themselves as being in a tribe at all. Believers within wholly Catholic cultures do not think of themselves as being in a tradition. Doesn't everyone live their way? Only when cultures bump into cultures and people interact with other peoples does the subject of traditions come up.

For 450 years and more, Protestants have bumped into or collided and interacted intimately with more people of more traditions—be they Jewish, Catholic, or secular—than have almost any other people on earth. On the soil of northwest Europe, the British Isles, North America, and outposts to which their missionaries and inventions went, it has been most difficult to hold on to specific traditions. In these cultures, people have led the least sheltered lives. A child could grow up meeting not only Methodists but Presbyterians, Catholics, Lutherans, and Jews. Few ghetto walls or sectarian shelters protected them. As such youth encountered each other, the edges of their traditions were worn smooth. What each held distinctively about being saved and being well eroded, blurred, and blended. Their heirs have had to be told that they are in traditions. They have had to be taught how to retrieve what might be helpful and healing within their heritages.

We shall focus on one of these traditions, the Lutheran, to see to what degree it is extant. What is "in" it? What is retrievable so far as the search for wellness is concerned?

PROBLEMS AND POSSIBILITIES
IN THE LUTHERAN TRADITION

Lutherans, who like to think of theirs as "the oldest and largest" of the Protestant families (it is the third largest in North America) make a good case study. When it comes to the issue of being saved or being well, however, most people are not interested in merely being part of a case study. Few care much about statistics or history. They want to *be* saved, to *be* well. They do not want to be human guinea pigs, but rather human beings, precious to God, valuable to themselves, cherished by others. They do not want to be read to out of recipe books; they want food. They will not be saved by the prescriptions they carry in their hands; they need the actual vitamins or medicines.

Lutherans are not exotic enough—as they would regard Mormons or Christian Scientists—to inspire mere curiosity on the part of non-Lutherans. Who would read a book like this about such ordinary people unless it might contribute to well-being? Most Lutherans themselves will sustain interest only if a book of information becomes also a book of guidance and therapy. Physicians who serve people of this faith would be hard-pressed to list their characteristics. An author has no right to bid for their time unless he or she might help discern clues that could be of use for understanding each patient a bit better, of discovering suggestions for improvement of their well-being.

The idea of a case study or guinea piggery should not, however, be passed over too quickly. People can learn how to think from cases they study. Those who are outside a tradition can learn something for their own well-being from a tradition of which they cannot become or do not even wish to be a part. As a Western Christian I could not, through sixty years of study or effort, become a good and true Zen Buddhist or Hindu yogi. For me to become one, my ancestors would have had to have eaten rice for a few thousand years. Yet there are *some* things I can learn from Buddhist and Hindu lore. Oriental ways of regarding time are different from mine. Although I cannot wholly adopt theirs, I can "think my way into them" enough to benefit from them, if indeed they offer benefits. In a world of bumping, colliding, and interacting traditions there is no point for people to hide within their shells. They can turn diversity into something positive by exploring traditions through case studies.

Although some non-Lutherans may profit from a case study, it is likely that the most faithful readers of pages like these will be people in the Lutheran tradition itself. "How can I be well?" is their natural question. About ten million Americans are called Lutheran. Up to eighty million humans share that faith name. A naive publisher would savor the potential market. A book that deals with the second most urgent question on Lutheran minds cannot help but be lusted for and fought over. People want well-being. They are in a tradition. Traditions promote well-being. They must find what is available in their own and put it to work. It all sounds so easy.

"Not so fast!" thinks the publisher on second thought, as she wakes to the realization that studies of this sort have not necessarily been best sellers. "Not so fast!" think thoughtful theologians, pastors, physicians, and other leaders. It must occur to them that if Lutheran lore is so helpful for well-being there must be a library full of books about it. Then they came to wonder where those books are. A trip to the library should satisfy curiosity. Lutherans have written and read thousands of books in and about their tradition. Almost all of these have been books about being saved. Their church tradition is nothing if not literate. It was born in the university, as a result of a revolt of an exciting junior faculty at Wittenberg, Germany. The Lutheran reform was very bookish. Leaders based it on the recovery of elements in The Book and of arguments from old books. They spread the movement through the new kind of books that were made possible by the invention of printing. Lutherans are verbal, even wordy. Where are their verbs about "being well," their words of good counsel on well-being?

A researcher who would answer such questions must stumble at once onto many problems that force the postponement of any ideas of help. Anyone who knows anything at all about the Lutheran tradition has to know that it utterly lacks healing gimmicks and devices. Its teachers have neither promoted vegetarianism nor offered guidelines on the recommended frequency of sexual intercourse. Lutherans, for the most part, have not avoided caffeine. The coffeehouse was proverbial in Lutheran Germany. The coffeepot animates the household in Lutheran Scandinavia, just as the teapot does in Anglican England or the chocolate pot does in Reformed Holland. (Though perhaps, on second thought, the coffeehouse and coffeepot *are* part of "well-being" on Lutheran landscapes!) Lutherans, including their pastors, have smoked. Some still do. If they stop, it is more likely as a response to U.S. Surgeon General reports than to Lutheran theology. Most Lutheran churches have not passed ordinances against the drinking of alcoholic beverages. They have no official lists of calisthenic exercises, no diet control mechanisms. There are no Lutheran vitamins or "possibility philosophies" on the well-being market. Physicians are not familiar with any shelf of Lutheran medical texts.

This absence of products and devices, however, does not demoralize Lutherans. They get their words from what they hear as the Word and in words. When they are interested as Christians in saving someone, they do not give an antidote for ingested poison or throw a lifeline because the person is drowning. (Of course, they should be ready to perform these acts if internal poison and external water are someone's urgent problems at the moment.) No, to "save" you, they will use words. They will tell stories about a God who made the world and who did not abandon it when the world rebelled.

Lutherans will seek to rescue others through a narrative about what God has done and is doing in the gift of Jesus Christ on the cross. Some Lutherans will reinforce the narrative with "confessions" or creeds. These are statements of belief that bring order to faith and to the quest for salvation. Words are themselves helpers, healers, instruments for saving people. The Lutheran tradition says that when the Word is heard and believed, something really happens, it does not *not* happen. Words are urgent. Physicians know the power of words when they counsel patients. This idea is not alien to them.

Then one moves from the sanctuary of salvation to the outer court, where "well-being" is the concern. There, too, a reader should not expect vitamin pills or diet prescriptions, but only words that inspire care or promote healing. With the passing of each year, more and more medical people are learning and teaching this idea: how one *thinks* about the body and its health or illness has much to do with its health or illness.

People who benefit from Zen may undertake some physical regimens. They may have to learn new postures or bodily techniques. Yet these devices only enhance a Zen way of thinking, being, and relating to reality. The books about well-being that you find at an American airport newsstand are usually the only tools one needs for a therapy, unless they are sold by a vitamin peddler to advertise his product. Reading, discussing, thinking, reflecting—all these become part of well-being. For such reasons the quest for the Lutheran tradition of words, articles, and books can be valuable.

In all those universities from which Lutheranism spread there are libraries. Wherever Lutherans have prospered, there are publishing houses. Shelves groan with their books. Lutheran thinkers keep producing even more on how to be saved. As for the subject of being well? Let me risk a claim that I hope some reader can disprove. In over 450 years, no book devoted exclusively to the subject in the Lutheran tradition has appeared or, at least, survived. I make this claim with the sense of nervousness that historians get whenever they say "never!" and with a measure of faith in the colleagues whom I have consulted. The project of which this book is a part includes researchers who have research assistants. Their computers spew print-outs, their book lists point to other book lists, and their footnotes have footnotes. Yet together we cannot turn up titles on "well-being in the Lutheran tradition." The second most urgent question on Lutheran minds has been treated very frequently but always incidentally, momentarily, or obliquely.

This book grows up in the company of similar volumes on well-being in the Catholic and Jewish traditions. I have considerable envy for their authors. A person can see, feel, touch, and argue with their traditions of well-being. A colleague who writes in the Reformed and mainline Protestant tradition and I must be content to deal with blurs, fuzzy sensations, and speculations when we treat our own. Are we like those primitive tribal people who are in a tradition but do not know this because it is too close to them? Certainly that is at least part of the problem. But if Catholics and Jews should glance from their tribes to ours, will they find anything distinctive? I would answer yes. And I would also maintain that most of what Lutheranism has to say about *well-being*, also in the physical sense, is an analogy to what the tradition says about *being saved*.

The idea of analogy may sound complicated, but we will deal with it simply. It has to do with "similarities within differences" and "differences within similarities." When two things are analogous, they correspond to each other in some respects, particularly in the way they work or what they offer. In most other respects, however, they are not similar. In logic, one who argues works on the assumption that, if analogy is present, at least two things have *something* in common. The two may therefore also have more things in common—if you think about it—even though they keep and display differences. Thus sleep and death have analogous relations. In both cases the observed person, the sleeper and the dead one, is in some sort of passive state. By analogy, they are similar in that neither has control over conscious brain functions. They are different in that one will wake to new consciousness in brain life after sleep, whereas the other will not awaken in the physical world after death. Of course, medically, there are an infinite number of other differences. To most doctors, in fact, the use of the image of sleep is only a poetic metaphor for death. It communicates little of a scientific character about similarities.

The concern for "being well" treats a number of themes. In the present case they include, for example, "well-being," illness and madness, suffering, caring, healing, morality and ethics, generativity or sexuality, passages of life, and ceasing to be. We merely rattle them off now, though they will be discussed in sequence as the themes of this book. What Lutherans have to say on each will in some respects derive from analogies to what they have to say about "being saved." Exactly what that means has to await later unfolding. For now, we propose it only to advance the argument.

The first word in any tradition determines much that will follow. Thus Seventh-Day Adventism was born at a time when Americans were beginning to learn health consciousness in new ways. Sylvester Graham, a Presbyterian evangelist, was spreading the word of health foods, including the "Graham cracker," alongside the Gospel of Jesus Christ. At the same time, others were on the circuit telling people not to masturbate or have intercourse too frequently. Still others fought the lures of tobacco or caffeine. Such Adventist founders as Ellen Gould White fused these interests with other concerns, for instance the Saturday Sabbath and the Second Coming of Jesus. They assured that wherever Adventism is present there will be a particular tradition of physical well-being. Something similar went on, of course, in the founding of Christian Science. Its first words are symbolized in the title of Founder Mary Baker Eddy's book *Science and Health with Key to the Scriptures*. All later words elaborate on these first ones.

Methodist founder John Wesley, in the family of mainline Protestantism, did write *The Christian Physic*. If they care to, Wesleyans can go back to origins and see what their faith had to do with well-being in the eyes of their first leader. Martin Luther wrote no work on "science and health" in his many versions of a "Key to the Scriptures." He devoted no books to "the Christian physic." So there are no "first words" to tilt his tradition to work producing book lists on well-being. All those writers of books on Lutheranism's way of being saved have had little to go on in the first generation so far as specific words on being well were concerned.

What was that "first word" of the first generation in the Lutheran tradition as a branch of the Western Christian Church? What is the basis for its analogies between "being saved" and "being well"? To answer these questions, we shall call on one of those Lutheran authors. In 1909 the late Einar Billing, a bishop of the Church of Sweden, produced a miniature classic translated as *Our Calling*. It is important to note that his, too, was not a book on "being saved." The calling meant how to regard one's daily walk and way, one's place and position in the world of work and leisure, one's morals and morale. If our principle can stand up, this means that he had to connect these "by analogy" to what it meant to speak of being saved.

Billing spoke only of Martin Luther, who is not the whole of Lutheranism and dare not even be allowed too big a part. Let the name "Luther" in these next few paragraphs stand for the whole first generation of Lutheran witnesses and founders. The general point about Luther and his colleagues, the pioneers, is of extreme importance for understanding this faith tradition. Remember also that what Billing says about the integrity of a tradition, the way its system holds together, applies as well to all other ones. What does he say?

> Whoever knows Luther, even but partially, knows that his various thoughts do not lie alongside each other, like pearls on a string, held together only by common authority or perchance by a line of logical argument, but that they all, as tightly as the petals of a rosebud, adhere to a common center, and radiate out like the rays of the sun from *one* glowing core, the gospel of the forgiveness of sins.

Remember that "the gospel of the forgiveness of sins" is here a clue, a code word, a signal of a rich reality that appears best in story form. Lutheran scholars use different terms for what it condenses. If they want to be formal and risk losing the ears of many people along the way, they may speak of "justification by grace through faith." Some may join modern maverick Lutheran Paul Tillich in translating this as "the gospel that God in Jesus Christ accepts the unacceptable." For the moment, we can let the gospel of the forgiveness of sins stand. If a person believes in this until it becomes the center of spiritual life, then by analogy and indirection the Lutheran tradition can have something to say about well-being, including about wholeness in the order of physical existence.

Einar Billing is insistent on his point:

> Anyone wishing to study Luther would indeed be in no peril of going astray were he to follow this rule: never believe that you have a correct understanding of a thought of Luther before you have succeeded in reducing it to a simple corollary of the thought of the forgiveness of sins.

Billings's own examples at first were rather churchly and churchy. The theory of the sacraments and the idea of the church, of course, spread from this glowing core. Then he moved out into the living of life: so it was also with the idea of Christian liberty in the world, or with the teaching about the call in the midst of it. Therefore, to Luther and Lutherans, something as "external" and "worldly" as one's call is "primarily a gift, and only in the second or third place a duty." Luther therefore "cries out to the farmer at his plow, the artisan in the shop, the servant girl in the house" that they need make no spiritual pilgrimage. "No, for there where you sit or go about your menial tasks, there you have even now everything, there you have God Himself. 'Should not now the heart of man jump and beat with joy, as he undertakes such works?'"

Well-being, like the call, is going to be seen as a corollary of the gospel of the forgiveness of sins. This will mean that "well-being is primarily a gift, and only in the second or third place a duty." Just as one does and must do much about the call in the world, so one has much to do in the matter of being well. Billing adds, "My call is the form my life takes according as God Himself organizes it for me through His forgiving grace. Life organized around the forgiveness of sins, that is Luther's idea of the call." So it is also of well-being, which is "the form my life takes," also physically and therapeutically when it comes to the matter of wholeness.[1] At this point, a point that may disappoint any surviving seekers of Lutheran potions or diet prescriptions, we have to leave the analogies and corollaries in mid-air or mid-paragraph, to await later development. Billing's statements press a second preliminary theme on us. By mentioning the words of Martin Luther he points to only the first and oldest, albeit the most mountainous of the hills to be mined in the Lutheran tradition. If we are looking for gold, we have to know what the larger landscape is. We need some sort of treasure map to use for guidance and to discern limits.

When people speak of well-being within the Lutheran tradition, they show little interest in events, moments, or clues to well-being that just happen to have been left by someone who happened to be Lutheran. We have a marvelous example to discipline imaginations in the case of medical pioneer Theophrastus Bombastus von Hohenheim, known in the history of medicine as Paracelsus. Ten years to the day younger than Martin Luther, Paracelsus also spent time at the universities that Luther knew: Leipzig and Wittenberg. He was a high-level dropout at both. Like Luther, this physician wrote in German, not Latin, in order to reach the people. He rejected medieval scholastic wisdom, as did Luther. Ten years after Luther posted theses about spirituality, Paracelsus posted his own about medicine. Like Luther, he burned the books of those with whom he disagreed in an act of defiance. Naturally, people called him "a Medical Luther."

Paracelsus bombastically separated himself from such confusions. "Why do you call me a Medical Luther? . . . I leave it to Luther to defend what he says, and I will be responsible for what I say. That which you wish to Luther, you wish also to me; you wish us both in the fire." This scorn is still in place. Mere coincidence of events or the sharing of a name does not qualify someone for being a mentor on well-being in the Lutheran tradition. We are not interested in a statement on medicine that happened to be delivered by a Lutheran. All that concerns us is when someone concerned with wellness acts out of or upon impulses, notions, ideas, teachings, or habits that manifestly belong to the Lutheran tradition.

When people appeal to the tradition, with or without good cause, they have to be taken seriously. When someone unwittingly also draws on that tradition, as innocently as did the unaware man who, by speaking, drew on the tradition of prose, he must come into our scope. When a story out of medical history or the search for health shows a behavior pattern characteristic of those we discern as being distinctive on Lutheran soil, our periscope has to turn toward its traces.

LUTHERAN DISTINCTIVES AND LUTHER

What is *distinctive* of Lutheran tradition? *Distinctive* is a key word. There can be little interest here in what is unique, a monopoly claimed by Lutherans. Few things in the lore of well-being are the monopoly of anyone. No religion I know of other than Jehovah's Witnesses reads scripture in such a way that blood transfusions are forbidden. No doubt, however, research assistants with their computers could find someone else to rob even Jehovah's Witnesses of this uniqueness and leave them being merely distinctive. If that happens in the green wood of an exotic religion, what can we expect to find unique in the dry wood of Lutheranism? It looks so familiar and ordinary on the landscape of mainline Protestantism.

One of the best ways to think of "distinctiveness" instead of "uniqueness" in Lutheran matters is to recall the brusque answer a Lutheran editor, G. Elson Ruff, gave a *Look* magazine interviewer to the question "Do Lutherans believe theirs is the only true religion?" He said, "Yes, but they don't believe they are the only ones who have it." They have no monopoly on God the Creator, on Jesus Christ, or on the gospel of the forgiveness of sins. They believe that their view of the faith is a corollary of that version of the gospel in a specially consistent way. Nevertheless, they find many other Christians being more loyal to it than many legalistic Lutherans.

The *Look* editor also asked a question we must pose about the roots of the tradition: "Do Lutherans worship Martin Luther?" Ruff said, "Luther had faults. . . . He made . . . unfortunate compromises, which nobody defends today. . . . Lutherans deeply respect Martin Luther. . . . Every year, Lutheran scholars write many books exploring his thoughts. But nobody worships him."[2] Many of Luther's practices and ideas would promote illbeing, not well-being. Jews, peasants, those prone to alcoholism, those afflicted with work sickness, perhaps some spouses, and many others might suffer from them. Why bother, then, with this fallible, flawed, often violent and vulgar former Roman Catholic monk who stormed across the German landscape four and a half centuries ago?

A story, almost certainly legendary in the "not truly true" sense, gives a clue. It was said that two Hollywood moguls—William Wyler and Samuel Goldwyn?—were chatting about investments on a flight to New York in the

1950s. Wyler touted rare books as being a joy to collect, a boon to own for the sake of profits. Goldwyn had never thought of the idea. He was immediately curious. Had Wyler any recommendations? Yes. At that very moment a New York rare book dealer was offering an extremely valuable sixteenth-century Bible for a quarter of a million dollars. It would certainly appreciate in value soon. The men disembarked and parted in New York. Weeks later they chanced to meet in Hollywood.

"Did you buy that rare and valuable book?" Wyler asked. "I sure did," Goldwyn said. "But you gave me a bum tip, and I unloaded it as quickly as I could." "Why?" asked Wyler. "It was really ruined," Goldwyn said. "Some guy named Martinus Lutherus had scribbled all over it."

In truth, Martinus Lutherus, Martin Luther, did "scribble all over" the Lutheran tradition. One need not have been a Roman Catholic, or a monk, a German nationalist, or a psychologically upset and guilt-driven person to belong to the tradition. Sometimes people are in the tradition only by name and have never felt a thing. Einar Billing knew this and rued it: "Slackness is the hereditary sin of Lutheranism, and with the exception of Greek Catholicism, there is nothing more slack than slack Lutheranism."[3] The tradition had included people who expressed important disagreements with Luther. The believers did not always earn the right to enjoy the gift of forgiveness, since it came as a solution to a problem they did not recognize. Poet W. H. Auden wrote of this in a sonnet on Luther:

"*. . . The Just shall live by Faith!" he cried in dread,*
And men and women of the world were glad
Who never trembled in their useful lives.[4]

So forceful was Luther about his experience, however, that heirs who do not quite share it still have to reckon with it. If they do not feel guilty, they still have to be somehow aware of their plight. They are separated from God in some analogous ("similarity in difference, difference in similarity") terms to those that his views of grace pose. Thus, they may alternatively think of themselves as suffering estrangement, loneliness, unacceptability, or alienation from God. Only the shaping act of God in Jesus Christ saves and restores them. So forceful was Luther about his expression, however, that Lutherans who do not quite agree with him at least know with whom they are arguing when they deal with their tradition.

Luther expressed only the first word, the decisive word, when he rephrased and represented the gospel of the forgiveness of sins. It is as old as the Christian faith. There were also second and many later words, few of them quite as decisive. For the official Lutheran tradition, one consults a collection of writings from between 1529 and 1577, put together as *Book of Concord* in 1580.[5] These "confessions" are a means of expressing and defining that gospel. Lutheran pastors and teachers promise to be faithful to their expression. These writings have little directly to say on well-being. They do determine the boundaries of talk about the gospel for which Lutheran views of well-being are to be corollaries.

In addition to Luther and the Lutheran confessions, there have been influential Lutheran writers and teachers through four subsequent centuries. We shall pay attention to some who did have at least something incidental to say about well-being. Thus, in our own time, Lutheran leaders are available for interview, and some have been queried about this subject in the lives of their people. Those who teach pastoral theology have special reasons to spread concern for well-being in the Lutheran tradition. The people called Lutheran, just by the way they go about things, become documents for understanding the tradition. The hills in which we will find some sorts and supplies of gold show many different profiles against the skyline, many different terrains and colors.

UNDERDEVELOPED LUTHERAN THEMES

As we survey the landscape and the library, it is profitable, last of all, to speculate in order to help the prospecting reader: Why has so little of the gold been mined? Why have so few of the corollaries been developed, so few analogies made? I propose six partial answers.

First, Lutheranism is theocentric, God-centered. When it speaks of the gospel of the forgiveness of sins, it need not be endlessly fascinated with the biography of the guilty. Some versions of Christianity and some perversions of Lutheranism ask believers to be self-obsessed. "Look, God, I am really good at dwelling on my sins. I have a longer list of worse things and a better set of really bad emotions than that Pharisee over there!" In the Middle Ages this attitude was called "scrupulosity." This meant being fanatic about holding up the mirror to the self and wallowing in the horrors found there. Lutherans are very realistic about what is in the mirror. At their best, however, they move on from this preoccupation with the human in order to turn attention to the forgiver, not the sinner. Philip Watson, a British Methodist, wrote a fine book summarizing the Lutheran tradition: *Let God Be God.*[6] Lutheran writers, in this lineage, do not automatically begin with a string of books on human well-being and techniques for arriving at it.

Second, the concern for well-being is a kind of taken-for-granted element in Lutheranism and many other faith traditions. No doubt, somewhere there lurks a German pastoral theologian with a computer who can tell you that 127,493,612,202 Lutheran pastoral calls in sickrooms have been made through the centuries, and that a certain percentage of them have included transactions that resulted in better health. Lutheran sermons contain countless references to well-being. Lutherans debate abortion, sexuality, suffering, and dying along with the best of their fellow believers. Most of the living of the Lutheran tradition, however, occurs on levels that are not recorded or reported upon. Historian Jacob Burckhardt once observed that what really matters in most of history is not written down because it is so close to people, so apparently unextraordinary, so taken for granted. Most Lutherans include well-being on their list of their gifts and searches as Christians, but they take the subject for granted.

More humbling is a third suggestion. Lutheranism has awesome limits. Lutheran faith has not so successfully impelled believers into the world to serve their fellows as have forms of Catholicism and Calvinism. Lutherans often let the gospel of the forgiveness of sins be a private affair, something to hoard and not to put to work. Unlike the spirit of George Forell's book title on Luther's ethics, they have not made "*faith active in love.*"[7]

Frankly, neither have they done what they could or should have done to make "faith active in well-being," beyond what well-being has to do with being saved. Lutherans need help. There is little reason to shout, "Hooray for our side!" Indeed, one of the most important things for Lutherans to do while enlivening what has been inert in their tradition is to find the principles by which they can borrow from others. The Lutheran tradition is not a static pond but a flowing stream, not a pressed flower but a developing plant. There is room for new flow, new grafting on. If Lutherans understand who they are, including who they are not, they can better profit from others.

A fourth reason why there is less Lutheran tradition on well-being than one might expect is because Lutheranism is not a sect. Judaism and Catholicism are not either, of course, but they have their own reasons for presenting richer traditions. Lutheranism, among Protestants, has tended to "bleed off at the edges" into the environment. It is at home in the surrounding secular culture and does not bid its members to vote for fellow Lutherans or Christians. It does not ask them to buy from their fellow born-agains through Christian Yellow Pages. Art for Lutherans need not be Lutheran art or Christian art: God acts in the environment, the secular culture, the ordinary Yellow Pages, and all kinds of art.

All this has meant that in Germany and Scandinavia people acting out of Lutheran faith traditions built hospitals and designed patterns of care, but they took no notice of how these could remain a part of Lutheran identity and expression. The result is unfortunate since it diffuses the gift, but it is also fortunate. This feature allows for a spread of the gifts in nonchurched culture and for the acceptance of gifts from non-Lutheran, non-Christian sources. Among those gifts is the set of mixed blessings called "modern medicine."

One more hypothesis out of many possibilities is: it has not occurred to Lutherans *yet* to develop their insights out of their tradition. In our time there are new urgencies. Lutheran hospitals, foundations, theological centers and conferences, individual scholars, and parish programs give evidence that they are playing "catch-up ball." Lutherans were equipped to relate God to the human through an understanding of the gospel of the forgiveness of sins. They were often less capable of expressing relations in community. Alongside the Gracious Other there must be the gracious brother and sister. We have been undergoing a relational revolution, one that has many implications for therapy and wholeness.

Similarly, we are going through what in technical terms someone has dubbed a *somatic* revolution. This means that people have new regard for the *soma*, the biological body. Some may say that this interest grew on Christian soil because people have become more worldly, less eager for eternal life, more desperate about making things work during the "one time we go around" in this world. All this may be true as a cultural judgment, but it need not be true in matters of faith. Christianity has some sort of somatic view of eternal life. Its creed ends with a word of belief in the resurrection of the body. The Christian, including the Lutheran Christian company, believes that the body is the temple of the Holy Spirit. What does it mean now that we know more than before about conception and fetuses, growth into puberty, sexual relations, organ transplants, and brain waves? Lutherans, like other Christians, await fresh work on such topics. We are not at the end of a dying tradition but at a turn in one that is rich in undeveloped possibilities.

On such a scene, what can an author propose as a method for gathering material, writing it, and hoping that it may be tried out? At times it may look as if we are using a vacuum cleaner that merely picks up all kinds of evidence. Then when the bag fills we empty it and sort the bits it has picked up. Or, to return to the hills metaphor, we pan for gold in the streams and see if some nuggets pass into the pan and can be isolated. Later, they can be refined and shined and turned into jewelry or tools for those who seek well-being.

It is more important to connect Lutheran belief with Lutheran behavior. Lutheran books of dogma by themselves help us little, and snooping on the Lutheran trail without knowing what to look for will help us even less.

Suzanne K. Langer has written that people's symbolic behavior has roots that "lie much deeper than any conscious purpose . . . in that substratum of the mind, the realm of fundamental ideas."[8] The gospel of the forgiveness of sins may be one of the fundamental ideas so deep in the mind that Lutherans do not even always know when they act upon it. In the words of José Ortega y Gasset, they may be *creencias*, which he says are not ideas that we *have* but ideas that we *are*.[9] At the same time, Lutheran behavior may express the fact that Lutherans have picked up as fundamental ideas some that do *not* square with the one that should be central. Many members are out and out legalists. Thus they operate in a zone of confusion. Legalists can develop a kind of well-being, just as can those forgiven in the gospel. But to stand between or borrow from both and blend them may be to have the worst of both worlds.

We should note two key terms. *Lutheran* here means the tradition and community of Western Christians that derive from the experience and teaching of Martin Luther and his contemporaries. It has developed through many periods and cultures into our time. *Tradition* means that which has been "handed down" or "handed over," in this case in Lutheranism. The word may refer to the heart of the experience and teaching of the gospel. It may mean the apparently less vital and sometimes more trivial characteristic ways of doing things. Tradition includes belief *and* behavior.

Tradition can be a burden. We speak of "the dead hand of tradition." Traditionalists do not feel free to act in fresh ways. They must always return to the past. Yet the past is gone. No one can return to it. On these pages we have little interest in curiosities from the past. The Lutheran tradition as a spiritual antique shop, or even a refurbished Williamsburg or Dearborn Village, to say nothing of a Knott's Berry Farm, holds no lure for us. It is possible to be respectful of tradition, indeed even to love what had been long-lost elements. But it is not necessary to propose that we would have been better off "back then," or that we can bring all of the past up to date. I for one prefer the chances for well-being offered among the mixed blessings of modern medicine, hospitals, pharmaceuticals, and therapies to the shorter, insecure, painful life that people in Martin Luther's day had to suffer. If anything on these pages expresses nostalgia for the days before anesthesia was developed, do not trust it. If anything suggests that the spiritual lore and personal care known in past ages might inform our times of impersonal technique, trust that.

No one can speak with authority for the Lutheran tradition. If asked to do that, we should stand in the mode of Paracelsus, who said that Luther should take care of his own affairs. No one can speak for the whole tradition, because each is only part of the flow in part of the period of time. Lutheranism has no pope, no official magisterium, no body of bishops who can define and depose. Certainly no scholar or therapist can speak with authority for the tradition of "being well" in Lutheranism. This book is part of a larger project, one among many in a new generation. It seeks to be of help to people who are not only curious about their faith traditions but who would like to use these as part of their response to the gift of well-being that is from God.

As in all matters affecting well-being, these involve some risk. The risks are not as high as in those faith traditions that say, "Pray, and don't go to the doctor." Probably the worst thing that could happen in the cases where I may have said something wrong in presenting the tradition is that these pages shall not have begun to do justice to all that is available. Still, modesty is in order. Where something sounds suspicious or out of line, the reader is advised to consult the tradition on his or her own. Down the block is a pastor, teacher, physician, therapist, or a practicing lay person who has Lutheran wisdom to offer. From reasonable contact with colleagues in the world of health and medicine I have learned a modest but helpful counsel: when in doubt "get a second opinion." Out of the experiments with many opinions we stand the best chance of growing. Well-being is not a finished product but a process to which many people out of many contexts will have their contributions to make. We are only beginning.

THE WHOLENESS FROM WHICH WE HAVE FALLEN:
A LUTHERAN VISION

Any person who wishes to be well has to have in mind some picture of what wellness means. When a carpenter has to place a complex panel on a wall, he first draws a template. This is a gauge that makes it possible for the eventual wooden replica of this piece of paper to match its intended place. A garment turns out well if it matches an approved pattern, whereas it stands little chance of doing so if the person who sews has no image or model, if all is done haphazardly, stitch by stitch.

Being well, we all know, is a relative term or concept. "Are you well?" the physician asks an incurably ill person. She answers, "Yes, pretty good." She is *not* well in the sense that her terminal disease is being cured. She thinks of herself as being well because that morning she woke up without pain. Her children, she knows, are coming to visit her. The mail has just brought some cards that reveal people care for her. A nurse smiled today and the paper boy was courteous and cheery. Her church newsletter arrived with its reassuring notice that the congregation had prayed for her. She does not face any unpleasant treatment that day. Her mind is at rest, her heart is at ease, even if her body is wasting. In her context, yes, she is well.

"Are you well?"

Different standards come into play when a coach asks this of an athlete and a physician of a cancer patient. The athlete is in the prime of her life. She is aware of some degeneration at work in her cells. For years the young woman has trained. The Olympic moment has arrived. She is in tune for it and, after answering the coach, will begin to warm up. The model against which she is working is not that of terminally ill hospital patients but the company of Olympic athletes who have made heroic records before she tries to do so.

Many faiths draw their pictures of wellness from some earlier states of humanity from which, they believe, people have fallen. However religions explain what has gone wrong with the world to produce illness and death or anything else that makes them misfits, they picture an earlier, better "fit." Spiritually, they reverse those "before" and "after" pictures that appear in so many wellness advertisements. Before a person took diet pills he was so fat; now he is slim. Before exercising, he had few biceps muscles to flex for the public; after, he can flaunt them.

Not so in religion. The "after" of people now, in history, is a worse state than "before." The goal of life, therefore, may be to restore or aspire to some good features of the earlier version. What was the original, or as people sometimes say, the primal or primordial picture of the well human? To answer this question, faiths tend to set human ancestors in golden ages and lost paradisiacal gardens. The picture of what it was to have a body back then, to have been a human being then, is the template, the pattern or model, into which one seeks to grow on the path to being well.

Biblical faith, and thus the whole Christian tradition, does present one such picture on the first page of its scripture. Being well for those who dream of a return or a fulfillment could then mean something like going back, or going ahead, to the image of human beings in the Garden of Eden. There they belonged to the whole divine creation. They lived in naked innocence, unthreatened by death and with no idea of sickness. Mental disorder was not conceivable. Humans named the animals, with whom they were in harmony and with whom they shared a world of natural beauty. The Garden, alas, is now gone. So is the innocence. For some believers, however, to be well means to recreate that picture and live into it.

THE LUTHERAN VERSION OF CREATION

The Lutheran tradition shares that biblical picture but does *not* teach its followers that they can be well by yearning or looking for life as it was in that original state. In dealing with its view of creation, including what it means for the human body and mind in the environment of nature, as with everything else in this faith, we shall have to look for its corollaries to the gospel of the forgiveness of sins. Only thus can it be understood. Only thus, for Lutherans, can it be of help in their own searches for well-being.

In some respects, Lutheranism is by no means the most alert and alive of the Christian communions when it comes to discussing the idea of creation. Its founding documents, the ones that pastors and teachers employ as prisms when they read the scriptures or look out at the world, have rather scant references to creation. In the bulging 717-page *Book of Concord*, the official teachings, there are really only two places where the pioneers set aside chunks of space to talk about creation. Pioneers? We might even say pioneer. The author in both cases was Martin Luther, who wrote a small and a large catechism. From these books people were to get their basic instruction in the faith. Because Luther was the author, the catechisms were the most widely read of the founding documents. Their teaching was bold. Their words on creation have had enormous influence in shaping Lutheran views of creation, the body, and human care. They help form the template for any who would be well.

A Lutheran can say, "In the beginning . . ." when he or she opens the *Small Catechism* to "The First Article: Creation." Such first words have a delicious way of making their impact before people lose interest or, in the Lutheran case, before readers hurry on to the Second Article, which talks about how to be saved. Luther first repeats the beginning of the Apostles' Creed, "I believe in God, the Father Almighty, maker of heaven and earth." Then he asks and answers the question "What does this mean?"

People brought up on the catechisms will have seen the words often. Many will have memorized them. But since the model for being well is drawn from them, a careful rereading is still in order. What is remarkable in them is that this tradition shows no interest in a primordial state. There is no backward longing for a golden age when God *really* created, over against God's limping, half-hearted, fallible work in the only world we now know. Not at all. Creation is a "package deal" or a single process. "What you see is what you get" in creation: the human as he or she *now* is is the subject of any current thinking about the meaning of creation, any modeling for wellness. The catechism words are not in the past tense. They do not talk about a primal world. With the exception of one phrase, "has given"—which also refers to the "me" who now lives—everything appears in the present tense. This understanding is of unimaginably great importance for anyone who wants to entertain the goal of some wellness. The phrase relates to creation in the real world, not in a never-never land:

> I believe that God has created me and all that exists; that he has given me and still sustains my body and soul, all my limbs and senses, my reason and all the faculties of my mind, together with food and clothing, house and home, family and property; that he provides me daily and abundantly with all the necessities of life, protects me from all danger, and preserves me from all evil. All this he does out of his pure, fatherly, and divine goodness and mercy, without any merit or worthiness on my part. For all of this I am bound to thank, praise, serve, and obey him. This is most certainly true.

Winston Churchill once said that you can hear a truth a thousand times and still miss it. On the thousand and first hearing, it suddenly hits you and the truth becomes true. Perhaps that shock can happen to people in the Lutheran tradition who have learned these catechism words, have treated them as dogma, but have never thought of their therapeutic possibilities. Can this one be their thousand and first reading?

It is well to begin at the end, with the issue of human response. Here the person who is seeking well-being knows that some sort of response is necessary. We can picture a paraphrase of the catechism such as: "For all of this I am bound to take pills, see my therapist, support my friendly neighborhood hospital, buy and read the right book on wholistic medicine, and watch my caloric intake." That, of course, is not what is said, though no such duty-bound ideas are ruled out by the words of Luther that explain the beginning of the creed. They simply do not represent the proper meaning of the creed.

Lutheran theologian Joseph Sittler once said that what makes the Christian community distinctive is the fact that it is a community of *praise*. Other agencies possess mimeograph machines and committees. Still others do good work for others in the world. The Christian congregation does many of the same things as others, but with its members' arms open to receive the gift, their eyes lifted to recognize its source. The Lutheran pattern can never assert with too much vigor that being well necessarily finds one ready to "thank and praise" as first steps.

After the phrase urging believers to "thank and praise" comes the command to "serve and obey." Service and obedience flow from the center of Christian response. For this the key Lutheran line is the one that connects creation with the gospel of forgiveness. It points to the character of the

God who wishes my well-being. God does "all this [creating and preserving] out of his pure, fatherly, and divine goodness and mercy, without any merit or worthiness on my part."

The very ability to keep my body in trim or to help me respond to medical care is a gift of divine goodness. The believer should think: I may undertake fitness regimens that give me psychological boosts. They might win me certificates from a health club or the White House. To enjoy these signs is humanly understandable. The explanation of the creed, however, insists that the basic gifts of life, body, and nature come "without merit or worthiness on my part." They come along with God's basic gift to me, the one that makes me right with him.[10]

What is most striking to people of other traditions is the Lutheran emphasis on the *now* of creation. Many readers of the Bible are tempted to locate creation "back there," back with Eden or paradise. They make much of the idea of *creatio ex nihilo*, the code name for the notion that there is creation out of nothing. This approach is emphatically not the center of the Lutheran theme. In fact, this accent is not even clearly stated anywhere in the Bible. It shows up first in 2 Maccabees 7:28, which means that it is in the apocryphal writings that Lutherans do not regard as part of the biblical canon. Jaroslav Pelikan, an expert on the Lutheran doctrine of creation, has traced the idea of creation out of nothing back to Theophilus of Antioch in the latter part of the second century of the common era.[11]

This understanding does not mean that Lutherans do not believe in creation out of nothing. They simply have little use for it when they talk about well-being. They need it only in order to underscore their faith that God makes the world out of spontaneous and free acts, "for the sport of it," as a psalm suggests when it refers to such creatures as the Leviathan, who rolls in the great waters. Such believers also need it to show that all things that exist, along with "me," are *derived* beings. They do not have life of their own apart from a shaping God. Both of these notions should help one be well, since divine spontaneity and freedom remain liberating. Meanwhile, human dependency on the part of those who praise and give thanks breeds its own kind of freedom from care. That is as far as the concept of creation out of nothing need carry those who speak of it.

If a person wants to be well, however, the greater weight falls on a parallel idea, *creatio continua*, which is so strong in the creed. God creates by being in the process of moving creation from chaos to cosmos or order. Originally, there was only *tohuvebohu*, the chaos that threatens and then promises. God thereupon moved to create order and is always in motion to keep doing so. *Today* the process is going on. God "has created me and all that exists." That *and* is almost too weak. In Latin it is *cum* and in German it is *samt*. God has made me "along with" all that exists. I am in the midst of universes afar and nature near. My destiny is linked to that of a creation in which everything is under divine control—herbs and medicinal agents, ores for metals that become part of technology, and ideas that live in medical schools.

God, further, "has given me *and still sustains*" my body and soul, says the catechism. Whoever thinks this phrase is stated merely to make the paragraph inclusive, to help the believer hurry past "body" to "soul," will urgently read on. This, we are told, means "my limbs and senses, my reason and all the faculties of mind." Bodily presence is by itself a sign that God keeps on creating. Then follow the physical realities of "food and clothing, house and home, family and property," all of which are part of well-being. As for health and medicine, God provides the necessities of life "daily and abundantly." And to address those who are ill, God "protects me from all danger, and preserves me from all evil."

The *Large Catechism* goes into more detail, but basically it reinforces the same theme. Now the question is: what does it mean to believe in a Creator? Again and instantly, the *Large Catechism* hurries past creation "back then," out of nothing, in the primordial world of a golden age or an Eden. It locates everything in "me," in the present time, in my body and in the midst of nature.

> I hold and believe that I am a creature of God; that is, that he has given and constantly sustains my body, soul, and life, my members great and small, all the faculties of my mind, my reason and understanding, and so forth; my food and drink, clothing, means of support, wife [husband] and child, servants, house and home, etc. Besides, he makes all creation help provide the comforts and necessities of life—sun, moon, and stars in the the heavens, day and night, air, fire, water, the earth and all that it brings forth, birds and fish, beasts, grain and all kinds of produce.

Then come the words that locate medical care:

> Moreover, he gives all physical and temporal blessings—good government, peace, security. Thus we learn from this article that none of us has his life of himself, or anything else that has been mentioned here or can be mentioned, nor can he by himself preserve any of them, however small and unimportant. All this is comprehended in the word "Creator."

With eyes wide open to dangers, the believer acknowledges that God "daily guards and defends us against every evil and misfortune, warding off all sorts of danger and disaster." The picture relies on that of the God who forgives: "All this he does out of pure love and goodness, without our merit. . . . "

Luther's phrases can never work hard enough to keep people from boasting. If they really believed the creed with their whole heart, he writes, "we would also act accordingly, and not swagger about and brag and boast as if we had life, riches, power, honor, and such things of ourselves." To think thus is to be "drowned in [the perverse world's] blindness, misusing all the blessings and gifts of God solely for its own pride and greed, pleasure and enjoyment. . . ." Luther also cannot resist the climax that connects being created with being saved: God has "showered us with inexpressible eternal treasures through his Son and the Holy Spirit. . . ."[12]

Well-being, then, is a gift that occurs to any creature who with praise and thanks, service and obedience, acknowledges the hand of a loving Creator. All this occurs in the situation of the human being placed in the midst of nature. Being well necessarily involves an understanding of nature and science. For the Lutheran understanding, one goes back here again to the man who "scribbled all over" the tradition, Luther himself. Of course, a reader cannot expect to find there modern attitudes toward natural science. Luther was born in the Renaissance generations during which whole new levels of mystery and mastery were being discovered. He no doubt wrote some foolish things about the universe. A few years from now, whoever will look back on what theologians and others say about the subject today will also smile over their ignorance. If Luther was not a natural scientist, however, his picture of the world was still open to science. The seeker of well-being within the modern hospital world does not have to close the sanctuary door, does not step into a profane world when moving from belief to science.

The German scholar Heinrich Bornkamm, in his book *Luther's World of Thought*, has traced many of Luther's views of nature and early science and found that the reformer was anything but a simple complicator of life for those who wanted to follow Copernicus. That scientist was then unsettling people by refusing to locate the earth at the center of the universe. Luther's view of nature begins, as does the scientist's , with a sense of wonder. The year Luther died he wrote inside a book of Pliny, "All creation is the most beautiful book of the Bible; in it God has described and portrayed Himself." Again and again Luther, in the spirit of the Psalms, invites believers to look at the body and bodily processes in such a light. He writes of the creation that *now* exists, not about some lost primordial Eden. Clouds, mountains, thunder, dew, and daybreak—all are signs of divine activity *now*. "The red morning sky [*aurora*] itself resembles the comforting, joyful proclamation of the Gospel." This we learn without surprise after having read Einar Billing on how *all* teaching proceeds from the gospel's glowing core.

If well-being implies that a person must be situated in nature, Luther is helpful. Although, unlike Saint Francis, he did not preach *to* the birds, he preached *about* them constantly. The birds are like living saints, flying hither and yon but merrily letting God provide for them. The therapeutic hint in all this is clear. When concern for human health and wellness comes in the form of worries that cloud the believers' minds, they are to ask: is this dark thought I am having one that deals with *today*, or is it about some vague future? Those who have recited the creed and who know about the character of God must systematically clear their minds of thoughts about future days. Is God, the God of the birds, also active in caring and preserving *now*, giving strength for *this* day?

Nature, in this context, is to be loved for its own sake. It is also a signal of God's deeply hidden wisdom as well as for its own purposes. Modern physicians or medical researchers remain on the trajectory Luther earlier proposed. They may see that much is still "secret activity in nature. And whoever is able to apply this performs more wondrous deeds than those who did not possess this skill." Luther, Bornkamm says, specifically connected this passion for inquiry to the pursuit of medical knowledge and skill. Such sciences are "based on this knowledge of associations and interrelationships, i.e., the function of each single particle in the whole of nature." The Lutheran tradition at its best has retained this sense of wholeness and interrelation within nature. It helps provide a charter for modern medicine.

The search for being well evokes a sense of curiosity and wonder, a sense that Luther wanted to scribble all over the early pages of the tradition that came to bear his name. He was benumbed by the fact that people took physical wonders for granted. "If an egg were no familiar sight to us and someone brought us one from Calcutta, how astounded we would be!" And: "We possess such beautiful creatures; but we pay little attention to them, because they are so common." Once more: "If you really examined a kernel of grain thoroughly, you would die of wonderment." The Psalms teach believers to take delight in God's creatures, since they are "so wondrously fashioned and so beautifully coordinated." Only "faith and the spirit" pay full attention to these.

Luther applied such ideas to human generativity. He thus provided clues to the concepts of well-being that begin in sexuality and child bearing:

> If God created all other women and children of bone, as He did Eve, and but one woman were able to bear children, I maintain that the whole world, kings and lords, would worship her as a divinity. But now that every woman is fruitful, it passes for nothing. If a magician could make a live eye, one able to see for the distance of a yard—God help us, what a lord he would become on earth!

Only the righteous saw all this, Luther thought. In a startling and most important passage he shows how the sense of being well contrasts with being ill. Of believers, he writes:

> For whenever they behold a work of God, they imagine how conditions would be without it. Death ennobles life, darkness praises the sun, hunger kisses the precious bread, sickness teaches the meaning of health, etc. The word "not" prompts them to praise the "being" [*Wesen*], and this implies that they search, explore, and ponder the works of the Lord, esteem them, and imagine what the world would be like if these works had not been created. Then they rejoice over them and behold them as real miracles.

Luther, because of his hurry to speak the gospel, often comes in second to the humanists of his time when it comes to giving attention to the value of what it is to be human. Yet he chided both them and the papacy for failing to locate the human in nature. Luther's rival back then was the great scholar Desiderius Erasmus. This humanist supreme remained a celibate within Catholic orders. Luther taunts:

> We are now living in the dawn of the future life; for we are beginning to regain a knowledge of the creation, a knowledge we had forfeited by the fall of Adam. Now we have a correct view of the creatures, more so, I suppose, than they have in the papacy. Erasmus does not concern himself with this, it interests him little how the fetus is made, formed, and developed in the womb. Thus he also fails to prize the excellency of the state of marriage. But by God's mercy we can begin to recognize His wonderful works and wonders. . . . All this is ignored by Erasmus. He looks at the creatures as a cow stares at a new gate.

The Lutheran tradition, we hasten to point out, also includes less wondrous notes. Luther's colleague and disciple Philip Melanchthon mentally stayed back in the world of astrology about which Luther had been so uneasy and against which he stormed. Luther had wanted people to be open-eyed and full of wonder about nature. Melanchthon relied instead on the natural system of Aristotle, which Luther often despised. Lutherans in the Melanchthonian line began to try to work out systems that harmonized nature or science with faith. Bornkamm sees a real "fall" in this move. He pleads for a recovery of Luther's deposit:

> A punier generation again preached a God humanly conceived and far removed from the earth, who had, to be sure, once upon a time laid out His garden of creation and perhaps still occasionally manifests an interest in it. . . . Until far into modern times an uncertainty and indecision devoid of the magnificent freedom once displayed by Luther prevailed in Protes-

tant thinking on questions of nature. His rich bequest to posterity had
been dissipated. And when the modern view of nature insistently rapped
at the church's and theology's door for admittance, there was no one who
ventured to reach for the treasure that lay at hand in Luther's views for a
true approach to the modern concept.[13]

If we discount the enthusiasm that Bornkamm the disciple shows for Luther, there still remains enough of his basic theme. Creation now has less to
do with an ancient Garden and more with continuing activity in the back-
yard and the bedroom. The basic attitude toward science is not one that di-
minishes nature and takes it captive in a system, but instead approaches it
with wonder and curiosity. At the heart is a wholistic view. "It is the whole
man who loves purity, and the same whole man is excited by evil lusts. . . .
The glorious thing about God's grace is that it makes us enemies of our own
selves."

This concept of wholeness, Bornkamm argues in another book, is urgent
for an understanding of being well:

> This insight of Luther into the wholeness of man was also a psychological
> discovery of the highest importance over against the ancient attempts to
> divide man into body and soul or body, mind, and soul. The self is always
> inseparably one, but the self can also be set in rebellion, in rebellion
> against itself. . . . [God] no longer regards the past, he cancels it out as we
> are never allowed to do, he forgives it all. To believe this, to let this light
> of the gospel into our hearts—this is the beginning of the new life. Then
> the gifts which God has furnished us take on new meaning and power. . . .
> In [God's] gracious eyes, which look at us in the face of Christ, we are
> again what he wanted to make of us: a new creature Adam as God thought
> of him.[14]

Lutheranism almost immediately began to lose Luther's sense of freedom in relation to the body, nature, and science. Even the very conservative modern Luther scholar Werner Elert admits this. The scholars after
Luther give the impression "that . . . Lutheranism in general is helplessly
enmeshed in a philosophy of life that is at the brink of death and is strug-
gling convulsively for air." Lutheranism, Elert wrote, shared this "en-
meshment" with contemporary Catholicism and Calvinism. But in Lutheranism, he insists, "the fact that the church limits itself, in Luther's
sense, to the preaching of the Gospel had to result in complete freedom of
research and complete freedom of teaching in the field of natural science."

At the same time, Luther's view allowed one to be free from the binding character of the latest findings in natural science. Luther's "belief in
God . . . is the opposite of every form of pluralism. It presupposes the unity

of life and the interlacement of life in the world as a whole. In this respect it is unconditionally related to the modern philosophy of life." All this has an obvious bearing on modern understandings of bodily well-being.[15]

Many official Lutheran teachings written in the *Book of Concord*, after the *Small* and the *Large Catechism*, appeared during the twilight years. Behind were Luther's dynamic, wholistic, and wondrous approaches to nature, science, and the body. Ahead came the development of the more drab, systematic, enmeshing, and binding scholastic views. We should not expect to see the original views developed. Nor were they. The later Lutheran confessions hurry to connect creation with the gospel of forgiveness. But they then drop the subject of creation. Yet a reader can glean from these writings at least one important insight on this subject.

Another conservative modern scholar, Edmund Schlink, poses the question that stands behind this chapter: does the Lutheran tradition's view of well-being call people back to an original state of perfection? "What in this present world is to be acknowledged as 'in accordance with creation'? That which is 'original'? That which is 'natural'? The healthy? The orderly? Is this, at the same time, the good?" The answers to such questions are remarkable. The words about creation immediately go on to say, "I am a creature of God." It is *fallen* humanity, the creature of today, who is involved. "God is our Creator beyond sin and the fall. . . . Accordingly, the very concept of creation itself contains the insight that it is by no means a mere matter of course when God permits his fallen creature to go on living." Schlink asks, "Did God, then, create sinful man? No. But man even in sin and in spite of sin is altogether God's creature." Elsewhere, the Lutheran charter writings add, "Scripture testifies not only that God created human nature before the fall, but also that after the fall human nature is God's creature and handiwork." The search for well-being does not lead back to Eden, to a primal state. Instead, it accepts in praise and thanks what God gives now and intends for tomorrow, a time that falls beyond present human care.[16]

To make a test case of how all this applies to well-being, it is valid to notice Luther's characteristic response to nature as it showed up, for instance, in play, marriage, and music. Luther was glad to read that the biblical patriarch had fun with his wife. "Woman is a delightful companion in life." The reformer possessed an ecological sense against those who would neglect, pollute, or misuse creation. "For God wants nature preserved, not destroyed" (*Deus enim vult servatam naturam, non extinctam*). Natural affections for family and friends, he argued, are not destroyed or corrupted. "They are not abolished through grace; they are aroused." He urged that "love and conjugal desire" were put into the human heart and should be acted upon.

Lutheran Pietism later introduced an alien element when it said, in Henrich Müller's words, "It is better to weep with Jesus than to laugh with the world. One will not find Christ when one laughs." Luther instead liked to say that, when God sees the happiness of married couples, "He laughs and is happy on this account." Luther favored innocent dancing. He thought fencing was a good physical exercise and that children "are the finest playthings." He had fun with his own. People were free to drink, though temperately. Luther thought brides should be dressed in their best finery. He could never say enough about music as an expression of continuing creation.[17]

In all this is a kind of anticipation of William Blake's celebration of "the Divine arts of Imagination."[18] Here is also the human as George Herbert saw him, "Secretarie of [God's] praise. . . . Man is the world's High Priest," representing the rest of creation, which cannot put praise into words.[19] Lutheran hymnody kept such an awareness alive even when its dogma and theology let the imagination of creation fall into eclipse, let it be clouded or doom-filled.

The Lutheran tradition, it goes without saying, is highly aware of the underside of creation. Nature threatens and produces terror. The body is subject to illness, the world to earthquake, creatures to the appetites of each other. The demonic pervades the world, though it does not have the last word. However Lutherans respond to questions as to *why* creation has taken the form it did, they address its present state in the light of the New Creation in Jesus Christ. In Christ "all things hold together" (Col. 1:17).

The Lutheran theme of wholeness and coherence over against chaos reappears when Jesus Christ is preached and believed. "All things" includes the world of research, medicine, and care. The last of the Lutheran confessions, the Formula of Concord, indicates how believers are to view the world of nature: "No one except God alone can separate the corruption of our nature from the nature itself. This will take place wholly by way of death, in the resurrection. Then the nature which we now bear will arise and live forever without original sin and completely separated and removed from it."[20] Meanwhile, we all have lives to live, wellness to seek, gifts to which to respond.

·2·

Illness and Madness:
The Issue of a Divine Role

In biblical, Christian, and Lutheran stories God "intends" wholeness and health for human creatures. Before the Fall human beings live in harmony with nature. No depiction of disease or death appears in the earliest lines of Genesis. The only form of the created order that people have known throughout history is marked by illness and the absence of wholeness. A yearning for a future state in which these will be overcome is understandable. The Lutheran tradition, however, carries few traces of nostalgia for Eden, a golden age, or paradise lost. Its whole energy presses toward an understanding of the broken and partial world we know today.

Bodily "illness" and psychic "madness" are characteristic terms for human speaking of this human brokenness. Illness and madness need not be constantly or chronically present in the lives of people, but they are constant threats to wholeness. The endeavor to become or be well occurs in the presence of pathologically jarring detours, barriers, or even ends of the road.

The problem of psychic wholeness or balance is complicated. Some therapists have questioned whether there is such a thing as simple "normality" or "sanity." The brain and the mind are such delicate realities and the behavioral elements that influence them or come forth from them are of such infinite complexity that science and faith alike have difficulty measuring what not being mad would mean. All bodily cells move inexorably to the end of each human being in history. So a mark of dying hangs over all the notions, attitudes, opinions, and ideas that belong to mental process.

What is familiar and profound often escapes us. Saint Augustine once said that he knew what time was—until someone asked him. So most of us know what illness is—until someone asks us. People know something of how it looks and feels and what it does. They are less sure of what name to put on it. Sufferers speak of illness when they are in the hospital, when parents jab thermometers under their tongues, when they feel impelled to take aspirin. They know how madness appears in the case of acute schizophrenia. Victims then act so strangely, perhaps so dangerously, that they might have to be institutionalized. Those near them call the psychiatrist: this must be madness! There are physical and mental symptoms that, when diagnosed, cause people in the healing professions and patients to recognize that, yes, they are physically or mentally ill. But what do they mean when speaking of fallenness from a presumed or intended state of wholeness?

Physicians and theologians fill library shelves with books about the meaning of illness without ever being sure of what it is, or certainly without being able to agree on the definition. The *Encyclopaedia Britannica* and the *Encyclopedia of Bioethics* include many entries on illness, sickness, disease; but their editors experience more difficulty isolating "illness" or "sickness" as such. The *Encyclopaedia Britannica* discusses the economics of health and disease without defining the latter, and that is that. The *Encyclopedia of Bioethics* has a fine "Health and Disease" entry, but it recognizes that both are "common but ambiguous notions." Explanations of what these are, we read, depend upon "biological knowledge, social structure, and cultural values," and these have varied through history.

Some writers say that health is determined by what disease is, and vice versa. That gets no one very far. The Lutheran tradition, they say, has used an *ontological* as opposed to a purely *physiological* description of both. That is, disease is "something alien and external to the healthy person," whereas physiology sees disease "merely as a consequence of disturbed functions operating within individual human beings."[1] If one wants to see illness as something that afflicts the whole human race, has some moral connections, and is open to theological interpretations, the Lutheran sort of view is necessary.

In the *Encyclopedia of Bioethics*, Guenter B. Risse succinctly summarizes a biblical viewpoint that Lutheranism also incorporated into its own primal understanding:

> The advent of Christianity reinstated the Old Testament concept of disease as reflecting the commission of sins. Confession and prayer directed toward the cleansing of patients' souls were the proper treatment. On the other hand, the New Testament included ideas and events that prompted some seemingly conflicting concepts of disease—disease is a consequence of sin yet subject to the healing of the spirit (Mark 5:21–43), a weakness which can be converted to spiritual strength (I Cor. 12:7–10). Under the influence of these concepts, care of the sick became a very important work of charity.[2]

Today, Lutherans in caring professions tend to mute this understanding of illness as the consequence of sin *in respect to particular persons*. A sense of acute guilt because of one's own illness can be a problem that itself demands therapy. As long as persons are obsessed with the question "What did I do to infuriate God so that God is punishing me with this illness?" they may fail to reach for the resources that might aid in treatment. The Bible already included concern for the general point. Jesus made clear (Luke 13:4) that tragedy can come whether or not someone performed this or that particular evil act.

Despite this humane writing on the guilt theme, the literature of Lutheranism, of course, does take seriously a person's responsibility for illness when a clear cause-and-effect relationship is present. It is not always ready to apply this courageously. For example, Lutheranism, for the most part, has had a tradition of "smoking." The parsonage in the past was often filled with pipe fumes. A concerned generation in the twentieth century found many of its clergy smoking cigarettes. The earlier literature sometimes counseled against excessive use of tobacco. Ministerial manuals offered hygienic suggestions concerning tarred fingers or told how odored hands giving communion could offend. But when modern medicine established strong statistical correlates between smoking and various illnesses, the literature only gradually changed. Editorials began to appear asking Christians to take moral responsibility for ceasing the practice. If lung cancer comes to the heavy smoker, the pastoral counselor is given advice on how to minister to the guilt. So it is also with alcoholism. Analysts regard it as a disease but also as quite possibly a fault. So it is with diseases related to overingestion of cholesterol and calories. There is no Lutheran patent on such moral concerns, but Lutherans have a way of bringing up the subject in order to focus the issues of sin and grace.

A folksy and somewhat tired story helps make this point. A Frenchman touring New York was asked what he thought of the city. He said the Brooklyn Bridge reminded him of sex. So did the Statue of Liberty. So did the Empire State Building. And on and on. How could this be? "*Everything* reminds me of sex," he said, thus pointing to what was presumed to be a French characteristic. Analogically, the Lutheran who looks at illness, madness, or any other disorder is going to be "reminded of sin and grace." Why? Because everything reminds the Lutheran of sin and grace.

The Christian belongs to a fallen humanity. If one conceives of the consequences in terms of the historylike narrative in Genesis, there would be no illness had there not been a Fall. Illness would not exist were there not alienation from God and a failure to live up to responsibilities before the Holy One. So we must conceive of the consequence in ontological terms, that is, as being descriptive of being, of the way things are—however they got there.

The Lutheran likes to work the subject of well-being to such points because grace is such a great focus in this tradition's view of healing. Rein-
hold Niebuhr wrote that there is nothing as useless as an answer to an un-
asked question. So the Lutheran has to get an ill person to ask the question
about sin. One of the favorite gospel stories on which Lutherans like to reflect in respect to disease is the case of the man lowered through a roof to
Jesus for the sake of physical healing (Mark 2:1–12). Jesus instead, or at
first, heals the man of sin by proclaiming forgiveness. Then, second, physical healing may, and in that story did, follow.

Other religions join Christianity in connecting illness with responsibility
and fault. Fran de Graeve, in the *Encyclopedia of Bioethics*, summarizes
the case for virtually all religions:

> Disease is a privation or withholding of something good, an undue nega-
> tive situation, inflicted by an evil or, as punishment, by a good and just
> power, or incurred by an evil deed. . . . A particular illness may be related
> to known or demonstrable physical causes, but there is always a spiritual
> dimension to that causality.

Yet the tie is not always individual. De Graeve illustrates from the Bible.

> . . . Sin and disease transcend the individual dimension: "The fathers
> have eaten sour grapes and the children's teeth are set on edge" was obvi-
> ously a common proverb, which Jeremiah and Ezekiel felt necessary to re-
> ject in favor of personal punishment for personal guilt. [Yet] because the
> good order of creation has been disturbed objectively, the whole of crea-
> tion is suffering the consequences.[3]

In the same encyclopedia an article by H. Tristram Engelhardt, Jr., offers another perspective. He opens the philosophical door for Lutheran understandings. Engelhardt ponders how important the medical profession
has found the task of naming, coding, and classifying. Historically, it has
been concerned with presenting various models of "what went wrong" in
the conditions that we speak of as illness or madness.

Medicine, seeking general laws, tests various models in different periods. "The meaning of the phenomena observed (i.e., the illnesses with
their clinical signs and symptoms) is reinterpreted in terms of disease
models." Today, he adds, "A great deal of contemporary philosophical discussion concerning concepts of health and disease is focused upon whether
their features are discovered or invented. Are certain functions natural, so
that their absence defines disease states?" Some theorists, he notes, have
said that one *can* specify those functions that are automatically a part of

being human. They can thus develop conceptions of disease that are not arbitrary.

Engelhardt, on the other hand, sides with scholars who believe "that definitions of disease and health depend upon value judgments." They therefore can be understood only in the context of specific traditions, such as the Christian, and cultural complexes such as those that exist in particular tribes or nations. A reading of the Lutheran literature through four and a half centuries suggests to a historian that this "value judgment" approach is definitely the case in its spiritual traditions.

The literature before and after Sigmund Freud is divided, Engelhardt adds, so far as the issue of determining the names of disease is concerned. "Concepts or notions of human illness, disease, and health are in part social constructions." Therefore, the philosopher notes, "there will be marked differences between the ways in which diseases are identified for humans and the ways they are identified for other animals." We shall see later what bearing all this has for Lutherans when it comes to separating the meaning of human death from the fact of death in nonhumans. Value judgments based on faith play a part in this separating and naming at all levels.

If I may translate all this a bit crudely and crassly: if you want to help "cure" someone, you have to get them to name the disease in a way that will match the names of the cures. Engelhardt argues, "For example, individuals who once were thought to die of acute indigestion are today found to die of a myocardial infarction (heart attack)." In such cases, a treatment to prevent death depends in large part upon the name of the disease. So it is also in the spiritual realm. To experience the "sickness unto death" that is caused by anxiety or guilt, as the Lutheran tradition often diagnoses it, opens one to a set of cures based on the experience of forgiveness. To see such anxiety or guilt always and only in the light of Oedipal or other experiences of that sort exacts a therapy that follows some Freudian scheme or other. In today's world, of course, these models, paradigms, and languages tend to overlap and become fused. Still, it is important to pursue the religious understandings to their root.

This point is clearer in the cases of madness and mental disease than in the more obvious physical illustrations such as myocardial infarction. Engelhardt reminds his readers of a controversy that has arisen about the status of "nonsomatic models of disease." Some analysts, amon. them Thomas Szasz, say that only physical diseases are real diseases, "while those states of affairs usually termed mental diseases are, in fact, simply problems with living." Szasz criticizes such a view for being far too dualistic about the aspects of the whole human being. At the same time, a theologically informed person will recognize that the naming of problems and cures has a more direct impact on the understanding of mental disorder than physical states of disruption or disease.

Those who doubt the role of "naming" in disease and therapy are likely to be brought up short by Engelhardt's most telling illustration:

> Masturbation, considered in the nineteenth century a serious moral fault, was also appreciated as a serious disease for which castration, excision of the clitoris, and other invasive therapies were employed. Individuals were even determined to have died of masturbation, and postmortem findings "substantiated" this cause of death. The disease of masturbation illustrates in part the effect of ethical norms on the psychology of discovery.

More positively, he adds as an illustration, "one may find . . . individuals advocating a view of alcoholism or drug addiction as diseases in order to recruit the forces of medicine in the control of these phenomena." Naming these problems "diseases" helps remove social disapproval from the individuals who are afflicted and can help others bring them toward wellness.[4]

The case of alcoholism calls for further development. The Lutheran literature on this subject is extensive. Beer drinking was native to the cultures of Lutheranism. Except when it developed under some Pietist controls, the history of Lutheranism has been rather beery. One historian, after observing how the conservative Missouri Synod of America Lutheranism opposed Prohibition as "directly adverse to the spirit, the method and the aim of Christian morals," nominated the synod "the most thoroughly wet denomination in America, or in the world, for that matter."[5] Treatment of people addicted to alcohol therefore became a Lutheran burden and specialty. Modern writers on the subject do not let the alcoholic off the moral hook. But they *do* want to see the addiction as a disease and not simply as a moral flaw. Alcoholics must take moral responsibility. They must live in repentance and under grace. The larger community, however, must not stigmatize the victims as specially flawed human beings.

The better case, one that allows a bit more luxury for examination because it has become less plaguing, is masturbation. Here the tradition has allowed for changes while remaining faithful to its fundamental motif of sin and grace. It changed because of new medical knowledge and new acts of naming within the healing profession. These forced new therapeutic and moral or religious understandings. Older religious taboos combined with now-obsolete medical "findings" had led to the development of models that found masturbation led to many kinds of physical disease and insanity. So widespread was the use of this model in Western and Christian soil that Lutheranism found little reason to assert distinctives on this subject. Masturbation was the sin of "onanism," based on a misreading of a biblical passage about Onan. It was always and simply the worst kind of "self-abuse." The literature dealt with this "disease" or "addiction" in severe moral terms.

Engelhardt reports on the changes that occurred when the laboratory and clinic could not find any cause-and-effect relationship between masturbation and ill health. These had their effect in the churches. The Lutheran churches did produce honest commissions and authors on this subject. Thus, a study by the conservative Missouri Synod noted that as late as World War I the synod's authors could speak of masturbation as "undermining body and soul and ruining health," as "stunting growth" and leading to insanity. In older days, one wrote, "The law condemns everyone who carnally knows himself or a brute or another person of the same sex."

This same synodical commission unearthed in 1949 a tract arguing that this immoral act "tends to enslave the person in his own vile lust . . . . There can be no doubt that it drains away much energy and strength from the growing youth." Thus it represents both a physical and a spiritual fault. The commission concluded, "All written opinions definitely condemn autoerotic practices as sins against the will of God." Back then masturbation was seen as a moral disease, which promoted definite physical illness.

Then came new clinical understandings. The Lutherans were not by any means ready to see masturbation as a positive good or even as a neutral matter. The act was still wrong, but now it was frowned on chiefly because sex in the Lutheran understanding is relational, an "I-Thou" matter. If narcissism is to be condemned, autoeroticism is certainly suspect as a sign of self-engrossment. Yet masturbation had been clearly downgraded in the catalogue and catechism of sins and diseases, sexual or otherwise.[6]

The consequences of such shifts in that most conservative Lutheran body became most apparent in the vicious literature of ultraconservatives. These rightists felt abandoned because the synod moved into a new therapeutic understanding while it was acquiring new names for the "disease." In *The Siecus Circle: A Humanist Revolution*, Claire Chambers professed to see a secular humanist conspiracy also at work in the churches, even in this unlikely church. Chambers subjected to review a sex education series from Concordia Publishing House, which had survived the synod's censors. The series, with volumes for each stage of life, came with the seal of approval of the synod's official publisher.

In commenting on a book by Ruth Hummel for nine- to eleven-year-olds, Chambers complains that "the author's treatment of masturbation is extremely lenient." Hummel had written, "Some boys and girls may worry about doing it [fondling their sex organs]. They may think that it is wrong. It isn't wrong. Almost everyone does it when they are young. It isn't wrong. It's just babyish." Chambers attacked A. J. Bueltmann on his book for twelve- to fourteen-year-olds because its "section on masturbation clearly gives this practice the green light." Bueltmann wrote, "Since masturbation is harmless, even when practiced frequently, you may wonder why I have written about it . . . ." Bueltmann saw the practice as a problem chiefly because people believe it to be a sin, thus inducing guilt in those who do it.

Elmer Witt, writing for ages fifteen and up, receives Chambers' scolding: "Nor is there any clear-cut condemnation of masturbation," a sin that Witt faulted chiefly because it produced "a sense of guilt." The book for parents by Erwin J. Kolb further "conveys the idea that masturbation is just a phase of growing up, and even rather encourages the practice. . . . Although the discussion later offers advice to parents on how to help their children overcome the habit, masturbation is never categorized as 'wrong,' but only as 'immature.'" Finally, for church leaders, Martin Wessler argued that "to the best of the pastor's knowledge, no serious physical consequences result from masturbation. But the consequent sense of shame and guilt can be damaging."[7]

This extended illustration of one sexual problem may seem to belong in a chapter devoted to Lutheran understandings of sexuality. Yet it appropriately illustrates change and continuity within a tradition. New medical knowledge forced an alteration, and humane counselors tried to provide a proper model or paradigm for a "disease" to match their cures. When masturbation was incorrectly seen as something that induced physical illness, Lutherans said, "Go to the doctor" and "Go to the confessor." When such a practice has to do instead with the relational understanding of sex and guilt, a subject on which this tradition has much to say, Lutheran counselors turn to the confessor and absolver, recommending their therapy.

These apparently meandering approaches, which may be ontological or physiological, integral or paradigmatic, reinforce an extremely important point. It all has to do with the theological naming of diseases, the special stamp a tradition puts on something. Thus, Lutheranism can never abandon its sin-and-guilt model in respect to all of humanity, even when it deals more gently with the individually diseased or mad person. The Lutheran tradition encourages ministry with medicines and surgery to the body when they are needed. It prefers to regard this support in wholistic terms, seeing illness in the body as a disruption of an intended wholeness that is a gift of God. Lutherans like to redefine the subject of disease to the point where their therapies, clustered around the concept of healing grace, can come into play.

THE VOICE OF ILLNESS,
THE WORD OF HEALING

Lutheranism is very much a religion of "the Word." It has characteristically provided little space for unstructured silence. Other heritages do more to promote direct or infused contact with God, mystical union with God on God's level, as it were; whereas Lutheran language stresses God's condescension, God coming down and humbling himself to serve humans. Thus "the Word" means that God is speaking, making contact, communicating. Jesus heals not by handing out the *mganga's* medicine or prescribing herbs. He heals by speaking the word, especially the Word of forgiveness or the word, "Thy faith hath made thee whole." The Word comes decisively in Jesus, but it is also heard in the voice of the prophets and is testified to in the Holy Scriptures, the Bible. Whoever wishes to locate Lutheran definitions and diagnoses, or the presenting of models in the field of illness, will find them clarified around the concepts of Word, speaking, voice, communication, and written scripture.

A canvass of a Lutheran theological seminary library will turn up hundreds of books on counseling in the face of physical, mental, or "wholistic" illness and therapy. Insofar as the authors draw upon the tradition and are not merely voicing current scientific models of therapy, they finally focus on paradigms of illness that relate to the Word. There has been very little interest—I can think of only one exception by a theologian—in writing about health foods. No Lutherans to my knowledge have written *as* Lutherans to prescribe potions. The attention is always on healing through the Word. This means that illness needs definition in the light of the Word.

Finnish theologian Aarne Siirala in *The Voice of Illness* wrote the best attempt to provide a theological understanding of illness in the contemporary Lutheran tradition. Siirala, who is well informed about modern diagnoses, particularly those centered in Freud, is ecumenically informed but also self-consciously Lutheran. He touches on writings of Erik Erikson and Norman O. Brown, who deal extensively with Luther and Lutheranism. Throughout, his accent is on an understanding of illness and madness through the concept of the Word.

Research always begins with a problem. As Engelhardt pointed out, problems in this case arise when experience does not fit existing ideas or when new events call old notions into question. Clarifying the problem is of crucial importance. For Siirala "the central factor . . . is the reality of illness itself, something which our everyday experience of illness shows to be most difficult to understand." Illness is always a stumbling block for those who encounter it because it shatters what we thought was true about life. Illness is so complex that we need handles on it.

Siirala focuses at once:

> ... The issue is this: Serious questions which demand answers have been raised by the encounter with the illnesses of individuals and communities in Western Christianity. This encounter calls into question essential marks of Christianity: the proclamation of the word and the establishment of community.

The author confirms the assumption that faith traditions have something to say on the issue of health and medicine:

> Christian communities—regardless of their particular interpretation of the nature of the church—are concerned with the ministry of the word, the word that destroys and the word that saves both individuals and communities. It is the task of *all Christian communities* to discuss the criteria to be used in differentiating the "right" from the "wrong" words, and to discuss the place of the proclamation of the word *in the total life of the community organism*. (Emphasis mine.)

They should use the word *word* because "in the encounter with illness a distinction must be made between a sick and a healthy forming of words." Both "becoming sick" and "becoming well" are manifest in such forming of words. Terms such as *psychological, psychiatric, psychoanalytical, psychotherapeutic*, and *psychosomatic* were not even available or necessary in the past. They indicate a shift in understandings and they promote newer understandings.

People have to make appropriate observations of reality and then direct their lives to accord with these observations and test them in their own experiences. For example, in modern times new perceptions have led us to seek words designed to overcome old distinctions between subject and object. What does this mean? Humans now live in relation to their fellows and to the environment in ways that shatter the older psychology. It was based on narrow concepts of natural science. People think in "wholistic" terms now. So did those in the Bible, though not many noticed this after the rise of modern science. Now "in the encounter with illness, the function of the word is of central importance as the organism becomes sick and well again." It is necessary "to listen to the forming of words in therapy," for they describe illness and "convey the message of disease to others." Words are the "sign language" we use to communicate with the community. Out of it grows communion.

Siirala says that *psyche*, with all its connections, is the most important root word for conveying symbolically the meanings of community. What does it symbolize for us now? Many listen only "to the voice of illness as it is interpreted by the therapeutic schools of thought which encounter and examine illness as a psychological reality." This language, however, is also very congenial theologically with the Lutheran tradition, even though it was formed before the Greek word *psyche* became a prefix to so many therapeutic terms.

The new therapies, we should note, came as psychotherapeutic challenges to historic Christian theology. Siirala reminds readers that his analysis comes "primarily from within the Protestant and particularly the Lutheran tradition," yet the word *theology* necessarily involves the larger, indeed the whole, Christian community. The therapeutic and faith traditions meet most creatively when theology employs "prophecy" as an appropriate form of the word. This term signals that "it had its origin in and is nurtured by a living, creating word" and not by a reference library about the Bible. *Prophecy* meant "speaking," saying, explaining. Individuals and communities in the general Christian or specific Lutheran traditions decide what they consider to be a constructive "proclaiming of the word in therapeutic contexts." Many choose Old Testament *prophecy*, which saw the universe, the cosmos, as sick. It is now a reality that needs healing. The healing has to have a cosmic dimension, must be the result of divine activity and thus "messianic." Illness is common and universal, so it has a voice that demands a hearing.

The New Testament takes these ideas over, as the healing ministry and word of Jesus make clear. "The blind receive their sight and the lame walk, lepers are cleansed and the deaf hear . . . and the poor have good news preached to them" (Matt. 11:2–5). The Lutheran tradition can easily affirm Siirala's summary:

> The texts . . . speak so clearly of the fact that salvation and the healing of illness belong together, that there can consequently be no establishment of community based on the biblical writings which does not face the question of the interdependence of prophecy and therapy.

Although there can be many different interpretations, no one can avoid the connections.

For centuries Christians stopped doing well with the encounter. Thus, although the Bible speaks of the power of salvation against illness, "church history tells of the isolation and persecution of the mentally ill," the separation of them from communion. For fifteen hundred years Western Chris-

tian dogma worked against therapy. "History shows that those who understood mental illness and were its spokesmen came into sharp conflict
with theological opinions; and the mentally ill were often persecuted by
churches." Yet, says Siirala, wherever the word of prophecy "heard" the
voice of illness, a more positive relation developed.

Whenever the word stifled therapy, therapists stopped listening to
prophecy. Thus, the Hippocratic outlook of scientific medicine, also on
Christian soil, saw illness as a mere phenomenon of nature, a disturbance
of the natural equilibrium. Medical scientists and Christians, including
Lutheran thinkers, settled for an artificial rupture; "the soul belonged to
the word of faith and the body to the world of reason." Churches and hospitals divided labor, but the mentally ill were persecuted by both. Both
Christianity and scientific therapy were responsible for the tragic breach.
Finally, however, "the voice of illness" broke through, demanding that
people of the Word take it seriously. Trends in humanistic and naturalistic
thought led them to change. Now once again a third voice, the theological,
is also being heard. The unity of humans with nature and in community
has once again begun to be stressed in the light of prophecy.

Freud is the main exemplar of "the therapeutic encounter with illness."
Siirala provides a friendly reading of the man who was often seen as a simple enemy of faith. "Therapy which encounters man in illness holds open
the prophetic perspective," although in Freud's case there was danger that
man be seen in isolation from the prophetic word. Still, the pioneer
psychoanalyst helped change understandings from the old "laws and var-
iances which have been observed in non-human realities" to a way in
which people again saw "the full interplay of all the forces of his
existence." Therefore, his therapy found new prophetic questions.

Even the atheist Freud came close to writing theology:

> The therapeutic encounter with illness has a vital inner pressure which
> leads to the situation we have called prophetic. In the encounter with ill-
> ness one meets destructive and healing forces in such a way that they do
> not seem to fit into other categories of experience. It is one thing to seek
> answers to the questions of our existence in terms of the categories of good
> and evil, of truth and falsehood, of beauty and ugliness; it is quite a dif-
> ferent thing to seek to understand our existence as a simultaneous process
> of becoming ill and of emerging from illness, as moving at the same time
> toward death and toward life. Our previous categories are not sufficient
> to encompass this understanding of reality.

Therapy and prophecy interact and keep changing each other's effects. It
would be futile, says Siirala, to talk of the biblical, Christian, or Lutheran

traditions as prefabrications to meet all circumstances. One's retrieval of these traditions is somehow always necessarily selective.

Siirala sets up the reader for a Lutheran case study as ambitious as was his Freudian one. First, he quotes a nineteenth-century Lutheran whose dictum was used by a twentieth-century secular Jew on post-Lutheran soil. Søren Kierkegaard once wrote that "Luther is a patient of exceeding import for Christendom." Erik Erikson used this claim to justify his controversial study *Young Man Luther*. In that book "history" became "therapy and prophecy." The illness and "madness" of Luther, and conversely his health and sanity, became a crucial subject for research.

Siirala develops an Eriksonian subject that is also urgent for our theme: " . . . Luther experienced deeply *the communal nature of illness* and strove passionately to express both his sufferings and his urgent search for healing. *Luther's proclamation of the word was born in the midst of an encounter with illness.*" (Emphasis mine.) This reinforces our claim that "being well" is second only to and is linked with "being saved."

Erikson was no more interested in limiting his study of Luther to "origins," in infantile issues as Freud might have done, than we can be in restricting the Lutheran tradition to *its* origins in Luther. Both must be seen dynamically, through changes in time, as each goes through what Erikson called an "identity crisis."

Siirala shows how Lutheran theologian Joseph Sittler in *The Ecology of Faith* confirms the notion of healing in a context with the Word. In Sittler there is also a justification of cultural and historical studies of a tradition. Sittler wrote:

> Every situation in which the Word of God is declared in preaching is a place and a moment on the river-bank; and the permeability of that time and place to the declared Word is bound up with the forests, the birds, the beetles, and the waters of history. From Incarnation to culture is a straight line, for the determination of God to embody his ultimate Word places man's relation to that Word inextricably in the web of historical circumstances. The Word is not naked, it is historically embodied.

For such reasons decisive moments, events, and persons in a tradition unfold new relations between therapy and prophecy. Luther, Kierkegaard's great "patient," certainly ranks as most decisive. For Erikson, both the old Lutheran God-caused and the Catholic devil-caused explanations of Luther's "illness" short-circuit the history. Luther claimed, "I did not learn my theology all at once, but I had to search deeper for it, where my temptations took me! . . . A theologian is born by living, nay dying, and by damning himself, not by thinking, reading, or speculating." Only theology attached to personal events and historical change can be what Luther called and advocated: a theology of the cross.

Few people in Western history, say Erikson and Norman O. Brown, have done as much as Luther did to prepare a culture for the therapeutic encounter. This was so because he had to reconcile death and life, wrath and love. Both authors trace Luther through his career to the edges of his "madness" and through his many physical illnesses. The exact character of Luther's ailments need not concern us here. What matters, as Erikson noted, is that when Luther was forced to speak his mind in public he confronted his own nightmares. Luther remained in agony because, says Erikson, "he was not a Lutheran; or, as he said himself, he was a mighty bad one." On the frontier of conscience, "the dirty work never stops . . . and the purities remain forever dimmed."

> [Luther] obviously felt himself to be the evangelical giver of a substance which years of suffering had made his to give; an all-embracing verbal generosity developed in him, so that he did not wish to compete with professional talkers, but to speak to the people so that the least could understand him; You must preach, he said, "as a mother suckles her child."

The word came in an encounter with illness that was experienced by the speaker along with a community. That is in part why Luther acquired a following, even if followers themselves had less fiery experiences. "Luther," adds Siirala, "found healing precisely in his sickness, not in escape from it," and there he found a new identity. God was not a goal to be reached but a way in the midst of afflictions.

In the power of the devil, added Brown, Luther emphasized what Freud saw in the death urge. "Theologies . . . which lack a real sense of the evil lack Luther's capacity for critical detachment from the world." The hope of Christ's victory then sustained the believer, the church. Today many Lutherans may find some problems with the explicit or, as some would say, mythological language of the devil and the Freudian language about the death urge. But both intend something similar: to draw people from the world of bland assurances and minor diagnoses to the world of radical risk and drastic cure.

The Lutheran tradition, never capable of living with the extremes of Martin Luther, revivifies itself when it sees illness and disease as part of a cosmic or universal disorder, a demonic attack as well as a moral fault, a social and communal disorder. Unless one can put the proper names on the disorder through the prophetic Word, the tradition has no resources for therapy or healing.[8]

No later Lutherans will experience the exact mix of Luther. Those who did not have the reformer's particular psychic makeup are not likely to feel guilt as he did—or, perhaps, to gain the same measure of gracious relief. It is hard to transmit one's experience. As W. H. Auden put it in the poem "Luther," which we have already quoted,

> " . . . *The Just shall live by Faith," he cried in dread.*
> *And men and women of the world were glad*
> *Who never trembled in their useful lives.*[9]

In Erikson's terms, the nontremblers were Lutherans; they were not like Luther, who trembled.

FOUR OPTIONS, FOUR FOCI

The Lutheran tradition has shown several sides when it comes to diagnosing and addressing illness. Many Lutherans simply are absorbed by the scientific culture of their day. They accept humanistic or naturalistic descriptions of disease and spend no energy at all providing a theological cast for them. Their physicians are allowed to treat the body apart from the soul or, better, apart from the whole. Perhaps some add a dash of prayer to their narrow and, perhaps even in scientific terms, obsolete natural scientific understandings. The faith they profess in such cases has no bearing on the whole of their existence, on defining illness or madness.

Another group of Lutherans may be more theologically minded, but they are individualists. In their understanding, illness is simply their fault, based on their own guilt alone, an aspect of their private punishment. Through a certain heroism of faith it can be translated possibly into good health. They pay no attention to the cosmic, universal, social, or communal aspects of disorder, to what Sittler called the "ecology of faith." Faith and disease appear to have no time or place. Masturbation, alcoholism, and indigestion are timeless names for unchanging problems. They pay no attention to either therapy or prophecy as these bear on the gathering, the congregation, the culture at large. Like the one-dimensional naturalistic scientists of their church, they will not be able to draw on all the resources of their tradition.

A third school appears to be more blandly conventional. Its members affirm Luther's experience and terms, but they domesticate these in dogma, practice, and quiet good manners. They are offended by the extremes in Luther's language and cannot learn from his experience. In safe and secure ways they may dabble a bit with prayer for healing and half-heartedly rely on doctors. They seek no distinctive understanding of what the faith might mean in defining disease.

The fourth strand, running from Luther through such other geniuses as Kierkegaard and Paul Tillich, have made genuine contributions to defining "the sickness unto death" and "the courage to be" in the face of alienation and madness in their own time. Their experience is not easily translated to people of less passion and curiosity, but the names they give and the prophecy they utter help determine life for others.

Whatever strands they all belong to, thoughtful people standing in the Lutheran tradition may well learn from philosopher Engelhardt and theologian Siirala. The models for cure do change, and with them also do the names for disease. Yet there can be continuities. When Paul Tillich says that "alienation" and "meaninglessness" haunt people and drive them to rely on the Ground of Being today, he is saying, for his day (and kind) a counterpart to Luther's word. For Luther, the experience of sin and guilt haunted people and drove them to God for forgiveness. Out of this, both meaning and healing grew. In both cases, believers had to be open to therapy, willing to learn from events and change, ready to fuse theology through their own experience, eager for a prophetic word.

To the Christian, the Lutheran Christian, smallpox, acne, diarrhea, depression, and epilepsy all appear as natural and obvious parallels or counterparts to what they are in the lives of other believers or unbelievers alike. So say the clinics and laboratories. One does not look for special Lutheran DNA, genes, chromosomes, or cells. Yet only those who say that nothing *but* medicine in its pharmaceutical forms has any bearing on these purely physiological problems would stop with that banal point. Instead, we view the person, the patient, as a member of a family, a congregation, a race, at this particular time in culture. Realize the divine resources for healing, which may mean God's word for addressing guilt or alienation. What matters is the Word that defines, does its own surgery, and brings its own healing. Illness is a result and a sign of what separates humans from God. It involves the whole of the person in community. Health and medicine in the Lutheran tradition address illness when it is so named and understood.

In sum, the Lutheran addressing himself or herself on these terms operates with four foci. First: I am ill because I belong to creaturehood, am a *member of the fallen human race*. If I am to be well, I must draw upon what God has done to change the condition of this fallen human race. Second: I am ill in this time and this place, perhaps as a result of a contagion, an environmental condition, a set of bad habits. I define this illness partly in terms that this *culture* and its therapies offer. Third: I am ill within this community and *tradition*, this way of telling and hearing a story, this way of listening to "the voice of illness" and of then speaking a word to it. I will get help from the form of prophecy that is appropriate to this therapy. Fourth: I am ill not only in the community of peoplehood, culture, and tradition; I am also ill alone, by myself. My illness learns from others and communicates to them. But it is part of my unique, set-apart, *personal* condition and circumstances. If I am to find or know well-being, I will do so in part because my physicians, counselors, and speakers of the word diagnose my specific condition.

Those four foci represent something of the complexity of being ill and defining illness or well-being. Yet they also point to several sorts of resources, any of which might aid in the search for wholeness. Standing within them, the believer experiences more security, a freedom to face what those outside the tradition—including modern therapists with their namings of disease—also have to offer.

·3·
Suffering:
The Theology of the Cross

A religious tradition such as the Lutheran, which makes little of herbs, potions, natural medicines, prescriptions, or bodily exercises, may seem useless to some people who are in quest of well-being. Yet when it comes to the *meaning* of illness and health, of wellness and disease, of pleasure and pain, such a tradition can come alive and have very much to say. People can endure any kind of *how* if they can endure a *why*. Of course, a person who is suffering acute physical pain wants nothing more than for it to go away. Yet if the pain remains, but there is a choice between finding some meaning accompanying it or *not* finding such meaning, the "well-minded" person will choose understanding instead of a chaos that makes suffering worse.

The Lutheran tradition comes alive and does claim to offer much on the subject of suffering. This does not mean that it owns a patent on solutions or has even a unique or superior way of addressing the experience. Instead, this heritage offers concepts that match its root claims of what being human is in the sight of God. Those believers who have reposed in the tradition's way of accepting interactions with God find that the Lutheran understanding is helpful. One says, if I believe this about God, then I also believe this or that about suffering. If I believe something specific about suffering, then I may find some beginnings of meaning and these can contribute to well-being.

LEARNING FROM OTHERS ABOUT SUFFERING

Like all sensible heritages, the Lutheran has profited from its exposure to the surrounding culture and to other faiths. Especially when it comes to a diagnosis of the need for finding a path through suffering, Lutheranism is free to borrow. At the same time, its thinkers pick their way over against interpretations that do violence to their picture of God, their experience of the cross, their perception of reality. On those terms, Lutherans can have little to do with pure self-help philosophies or with those optimistic claims that pain is an illusion or that proper prayer will necessarily lead to the removal of pain. Whereas the Pentecostal says, "It is God's will that you be cured," the Lutheran has to do a great deal of interpretation. God's will may be felt or known as one in which physical wellness is not forthcoming. It is, after all, God's will that all creatures shall die.

Father Joseph Fichter, in his study *Religion and Pain*, presents a virtual anthology of characteristic addresses to the urgency of finding meaning through suffering. Although only a few of these insights come from the Lutheran tradition, they provide a frame in which we shall present the Lutheran picture.

The Fichter collection begins with a gem from anthropology, the science of the study of what it is to be human. Clifford Geertz has posed the issue well. The problem of suffering is an "experiential challenge in whose face the meaningfulness of a particular pattern of life threatens to dissolve into a chaos of thingless names and nameless things." On those terms, if one follows the Lutheran way to the point of illness, doubt, or some other forms of suffering and then finds no further meaning, the chaos will only be worse. Therefore, "as a religious problem, the problem in suffering is, paradoxically, not how to avoid suffering, but how to suffer, how to make of physical pain, personal loss, worldly defeat, or the helpless contemplation of others' agony something bearable, supportable—something, as we say, sufferable."

The common human address to suffering has been religious. Sociologist J. Milton Yinger testifies to the commonness of that experience. Religion expresses human beings'

> refusal to capitulate to death, to give up in the face of frustration, to allow hostility to tear apart their human associations. The quality of being religious, seen from the individual point of view, implies two things: first a belief that evil, pain, bewilderment, and injustice are fundamental facts of existence; and, second, a set of practices and related sanctified beliefs that express a conviction that man can ultimately be saved from these facts.

Religion asks: "Does life have some central meaning despite the suffering and the succession of frustrations and tragedies it brings?" Another sociologist, Talcott Parsons, contends that "religion has its greatest relevance to the points of maximum strain and tension in human life as well as to positive affirmations of faith in life, often in the face of these strains."

Some suffering can be explained, but the sort with which religion must deal is inexplicable. If I know that pain exists, that some pain can be avoided, that I will have pain if I touch a hot radiator, and then touch a hot radiator, there is no special need for my having to plot a way through chaos. However, if a flash flood or hurricane in a place where these have never been seen as hazards wipes out my life earnings and all my treasures, if my spouse takes up with another person and deserts me, if my child gets leukemia, or if I become an overlooked but tortured "political prisoner" out of witness to faith, then it is necessary to reach for meaning. Chaos or despair are the alternatives.

Pain is usually at the heart of suffering. While one copes with physical pain, the spiritual side intrudes first as a nagging undertone and then as something that might well overwhelm. Geertz says, "The problem of suffering easily passes into the problem of evil, for if suffering is severe enough it usually, though not always, seems morally undeserved as well, at least to the sufferer." Here comes the God question, one that Christians call "theodicy," the act of explaining evil in the light of faith. Roman Catholic theologian Edward Schillebeeckx points up the issue: "Life's ultimate questions—and among them are certainly sickness, suffering, and death—must be answered in the light of the fundamental insights of our faith: otherwise the answers are not merely too superficial, but simply false." Schillebeeckx knows that human reason cannot fathom the roots of pain, that faith must address it or it will be deserted.

The contemporary Lutheran thinker Peter Berger brings these all into focus: "The individual suffering from a tormenting illness, say, or from oppression and exploitation at the hands of fellowmen, desires relief from these misfortunes. But he equally desires to know *why* these misfortunes have come to him in the first place." Theologian Albert Outler says that any serious person will "well imagine that he could have devised a cosmic operation less replete with frustration, suffering and indignity." Yet, not having devised such but still being condemned to the cosmic order that confronts people, they may or may not turn to God in the face of suffering.

Here Father Fichter brings his expertise to bear as he reports on surveys concerning how religious people deal with pain and suffering:

> First, there are some patients, even dangerously ill ones, who have no interest at all in religion or spirituality, and see no reason for developing such an interest. A second category is that of the true believers, the devoutly religious patients who seek divine assistance and have been accustomed all their lives to prayerful practices. Thirdly, there are also some patients, bitter after long years of suffering, who actually turn against God and proclaim themselves atheists.

In the first camp was columnist Stewart Alsop, who told of his experience with leukemia. During the crisis, with "a certain sense of embarrassment," he entered an Episcopal church, but prayer did not come. "The big bearded reality of my childhood is no longer a reality to me, which was why I felt a faint sense of embarrassment." Alsop remained an agnostic.

Of the third type, Fichter reports that suffering is not always a schooling for godliness. Some people *do* lose faith in its face. He quotes a Dominican anthropologist, Francois Lepargneur, to the effect that "the effects of sickness, far from making it easier to bring about a spiritual renewal, complicate the difficulty by weakening the capacity for seeing higher values by diminishing the person's interior lucidity." Still, "in general . . . we do not have much evidence from our interviews and questionnaires in church-related hospitals concerning sick people who turn away from God in their pain. . . . It is generally considered unseemly—if not un-American—to criticize religion and to find fault with God and his ministers." Therefore, some patients may be courteous to medical people and clerics though their faith has disappeared.

Fichter's second category interests us here. "There is much research evidence to support the generalization that the people who turn to God when they are sick are usually also the people who turned to God when they were healthy." Those who lived with an "intrinsic religious orientation," wrote Raymond Carey, were best able to adjust. If they held to a faith because it evoked trust and a sense of its being true, this faith stayed with them. They could not be latecomers to it, who used it as a gimmick or tool. Yet Fichter's research also qualified Carey's contention. Is it true that "the more religious a person is the more able he or she is to endure suffering"? Only 39 percent were ready to say yes; 48 percent of the clergy chaplains thought so, but only 31 percent of the lay nurses. Those who are at the side of people in their pain longer found this to be the case.

Although Father Fichter admits that his survey is preliminary and sketchy, it is a good cautionary word as we return to the issue of the Lutheran tradition. A faithful understanding of suffering is *not* an automatic instrument to make suffering palatable or conquerable. Instead, persons are faithful intrinsically, because the faith grasps them as being true and valid. Thereupon some surcease from suffering, some understanding in its presence, can follow. Fichter summarizes his two hypotheses in the light of his findings.

> It seems quite evident that the more religious a person is, or has been during the course of life, the more likely he or she is to turn to God in times of serious illness. The patient who has previously paid little attention to religion will not pray to God. The second hypothesis is that strong religious faith makes it somewhat easier for the patient to endure pain. For the most part, the health professionals in the hospitals we surveyed were not ready to confirm this hypothesis.[1]

THE LUTHERAN THEME IN RESPECT TO SUFFERING

Could it be that the heritage has resources that members of Lutheran churches do not know about, have not thought about, and cannot draw upon from their distance? Might suffering become more comprehensible if the "fit" between the teachings and practices of the faith in times of crises could be understood? Might Christians of other traditions be able to supplement their own by borrowing Lutheran insights? Positive answers to all such questions are not easy to provide, but we can contribute by assessing the Lutheran address to the somewhat universal religious problem of suffering.

Lutherans do not find "positive thinking" or "new thought" philosophies congenial. In these, suffering and pain are either illusory or they are able to be explained fairly simply. By acts of will and imagination, such as those of "the little engine that could," people are to think their way into success. Success means extension of life, removal of illness, release from pain, recovery of health. Never are such achievements the promise of Christian faith in the Lutheran understanding. Indeed, an almost brutal realism appears at the beginning point. Pain is real and awful. The search for answers is urgent but not easily satisfied. The questions will not go away. They intensify because this tradition makes so much of the spontaneous and persisting love of God. Then how do we make sense of it all? Lutheran theologian Helmut Thielicke poses this question graphically:

> In time of joy one can *forget* God because the moment is already "occupied"; but in suffering one can at the most doubt him: "Where is my God now?" This is why pastoral care is practiced in the wards of hospitals but not on the streets at Mardi Gras.[2]

Lutheranism cherishes the images of divine suffering and locates them at the heart of faith. This, of course, does not mean that it alone focuses on the miseries of the crucified Jesus. "Contemplating the passion" of Christ is not to induce grimness or morbidity. There is not much fascination with the almost grotesque visions of suffering of the sort seen in Spanish piety or flagellant cults. The meaning, not the detail, of Jesus' suffering is at the center. The Lutheran tradition, over against positive thinking, stays with the "why?" uttered in the Book of Job or by the prophet Habakkuk, to say nothing of in some seventy "lament" Psalms. Lutherans retell the story of biblical figures who ponder the mystery of illness and pain and do not claim successful conquest of these or simple escape from them through miraculous healings or reassurances. It does keep the possibility of miracle alive, but allows for no sense of failure when it does not come. Nor is the believer to focus entirely on it.

Along with evangelical catholicism in general, Lutheranism connects the two biblical testaments supremely through the figure of the Suffering Servant (Isa. 53). Whatever this servant signified when the figure first appeared—was it a person, or Israel, or something else?—to the evangelical this servant in the New Testament is Christ who moves toward a death for others. Lutheran theology, worship, hymnody, piety, and practice all issue from that move. God forgives the sinner, showing grace and love, because of the humble and obedient act of this sufferer for all. Lutheran scholar Heinrich Bornkamm argues that the *whole* of Christian living in this tradition can be summarized in three words: *love, work,* and *suffering.* Of the third he writes:

> . . . we use the word in its broadest significance, not merely the visible suffering that comes through illness, misfortune, or the death of persons we love. This is only the severest, most concentrated form of suffering. Nobody escapes it and we must constantly be prepared to meet it. But it is all the more important to know that all of life rests upon an unseen foundation of suffering, deprivation, and sacrifice. We all live by reason of the fact that men perform hard physical labor for us or that others bear political responsibility for us. When war comes, a part of the nation, to our eyes chosen at haphazard, are compelled to make the supreme sacrifice and others are spared. Without this law of vicarious sacrifice and suffering there would be no life. We do not really live our life to the full until we are willing to take upon ourselves that part of it that falls to us.[3]

The picture has grown instantly complicated. All suffering inspires a need for explanation. Not all suffering is specifically of the sort that identifies one with Christ. The suffering connected with sickness must itself be located in the larger background of suffering as a whole way of life. Suffering in the face of affirming the power of God in Christ is more puzzling than *mere* suffering. Suffering done with and for others is especially ennobling.

The idea that suffering comprises one of three elements of Christian life does not, in the Lutheran tradition, mean that one should go seeking it. There is no way to be saved by ascetic practices or by taking on suffering for the good of others. Nor is there special service to God when a slave mentality of humble submission to suffering under a divine Tyrant is the central theme of faith. Suffering will come when and how it wills. It never has to be invited. To make too much of it psychologically is a distortion of faith, a twisting of life.

From the far left end of the Lutheran radical spectrum, German theologian Dorothee Soelle has scorned a misreading of this faith. She is opposed to "Christian masochism," which she locates in the piety of Calvin. Soelle derides mere submission to God, especially in the face of all forms of suffering to which humans could put an end by taking action, especially joint and social action, against its root causes. Here the witness for the prosecution in Soelle's book is Freud:

> [Religion offers a technique that is helpful in offering a defense against suffering that depresses] the value of life and distort[s] the picture of the real world in a delusional manner—which presupposes an intimidation of the intelligence. . . . If the believer finally sees himself obliged to speak of God's "inscrutable decrees," he is admitting that all that is left to him as a last possible consolation and source of pleasure in his suffering is an unconditional submission.

Soelle can tolerate the simple confusions of popular folk piety. People with such piety overenjoy the act of suffering. She simply derides theologies, however, that allow for or even invent "as a companion piece a sadistic God. . . .

> The God who produces suffering and causes affliction becomes the glorious theme of a theology that directs our attention to the God who demands the impossible and tortures people—although this theology can, of course, show no devotion to such a God. There is little doubt that the Reformation strengthened theology's sadistic accents.

Soelle advocates socialistic and revolutionary patterns of activism to relieve suffering and feels that the picture of a God who causes suffering leads to a slave mentality. Finally, she compares such theology to the thought of Heinrich Himmler.

To those who hold such a Promethean view of faith, one that makes human agency all-important, there is not much point in the grand Lutheran theme that finds the faithful human being and God suffering together. Soelle attacks modern Reformed/Lutheran thinker Jürgen Moltmann for speaking of a "crucified God."

> On the one hand, Moltmann has carved out the figure of the "crucified God," the "suffering, poor, defenseless Christ," and criticized the ancient ideal of an apathetic God by portraying God as the "God of the poor, the peasants and the slaves," who suffers "in us, where love suffers." But this intention, this passion for suffering, is weakened and softened through the theological system that transmits it. God is not understood only or even primarily as the loving and suffering Christ. He is simultaneously supposed to occupy the position of the ruling, omnipotent Father.

This is the Father whom Soelle so detests. "Who wants such a God? Who gains anything from him? What kind of people must those be whose highest being see [God's] honor in practicing retaliation?... Why, in such a theology, should Jesus suffer 'at God's hands'?"

We reproduce this here not because Soelle has remained within the boundaries of Lutheranism's historic "allowable options," but because in several respects even her criticisms can come as valuable checks against misuses of Christian teaching, Lutheran style. First, there should be no seeking out of suffering, no ready welcome for it, as if it created no problems or provided for a special way of salvation. Second, Lutheranism's heirs should cultivate no "psychology of suffering" of a sort that induces a spirit of slavery, a desire for being dominated. Third, there must be an awareness of the part humans *can* play in minimizing some forms of suffering by the actions they take. Finally, Soelle points up well the reality that all pictures of God will issue in various sets of problems for intellect and faith. Those problems remain even after her "activist" and "anti-domination" testimony have been heard.[4]

In Lutheranism whatever one says about God in respect to suffering in human logic, some compensatory set of positives or negatives will balance each word. Why is there suffering? To say that God uses it always for punishing creates terrible problems. The New Testament itself addresses these. Why was this man born blind? Jesus answered with a question: what about the people on whom the Tower of Siloam fell? Neither the man nor the victims were special sinners singled out for punishment. All finitude connects with punishment, but to overdo the tie between my suffering and God's punitive spirit creates an abhorrent picture of God and paralyzes me with guilt in the midst of suffering.

The other proposals are also as full of problems. One may say that God *causes* suffering. What kind of God sets up such a cosmic and loveless operation as to create such meaningless suffering as a brain tumor in a two-year-old? What then is love? Or one may say that God *allows* suffering. What kind of person would permit the suffering of a loved one if he or she could prevent it? If God can prevent suffering, why should this God permit it? Most proposals lead one to see either God's power or God's love compromised.

Lutherans can never say enough about the power, about "letting God be God." Yet if they tilt, it must always be toward the love of God. So the most consistent therapeutic answer, from Luther in the sixteenth century to Dietrich Bonhoeffer in the twentieth, is that God *suffers with* the Christian, especially in the activity in Christ, and the Christian suffers with God in the divine humility of Jesus.

Professor Harold Ditmanson, in a paper delivered in 1982 to Lutheran bishops, set forth five or six such tensions. He said in response to questions that one could carry them in either of two directions. One is toward "Deism," the belief that there is a divine force or power, an agency that set into motion the cosmos, its orders and laws and forces, and then absented itself. There are normal cells in the body, but when they turn malignant no driving force personally serves as an agency to divert the body back to health.

Ditmanson's other direction is toward "folk piety," which knows exactly what God is doing. If it is God's will to turn cells malignant, so be it; if cells turn healthy, God willed it. The victim or the cured one and his or her observers can know precisely what this intervening will is. Deism satisfies a dimension of reason but does not square with the heart's experience. Folk piety can easily reduce God to a manipulated, controlled being.[5]

The "suffering-with" God is a concept that, without solving everything, at least avoids these two problematic extremes. It does justice to some biblical witness and much of Lutheran accent. Like all theodicies in the face of suffering, this one does not prove the existence of a loving God or provide a philosophically satisfying answer to the problem of evil. In the end, the Lutheran tradition does not worry too much about these questions because of its very modest view of what reason by itself is and can achieve. Lutherans speak of this as a feature of their favored "theology of the cross," their address to human suffering. This is the central note from Luther to the present. The framework for it deserves some examination and appraisal.

THE GOD WHO "SUFFERS WITH"

In 1518, in a debate at Heidelberg, Martin Luther defended a number of propositions. One of them set the groundwork for his whole theology. It was designed to prevent people from expressing "a theology of glory." Such a theology "has an answer for everything." It peers into the divine majesty, contemplates and theorizes (*theoria* is a Greek word for *behold*) what is going on in the divine mind. Then it expounds on the divine mind to humans. On those terms, Luther feared, people would try to go beyond their human boundaries and limits. They would try to be like God, to earn God's favor, to impress God, to be God.

At Heidelberg, Luther made clear that the cross of the abandoned, powerless Christ is the way God is revealed in the world. The cross is God's way of refuting the misunderstandings of the divine way to make possible claims of human wisdom and ways:

> 19. That person does not deserve to be called a theologian who sees the invisible things of God as they are comprehended in things which have been created [Rom. 1:20].

20. He deserves to be called a theologian, however, who comprehends the visible and manifest things of God seen through suffering and the cross.[6]

This needs some explanation. Luther remembers Exodus 20:33, where the Lord hides Moses in the rock's cleft. To see God face to face would lead to annihilation. God, having passed by, will move his hand across the cleft. Moses can then look out and see the "hind parts," the back, the posterior, we might almost say the buttocks of God. Luther insists that that is what one sees in Christ's suffering and the cross. That is all one gets to see or should want to see. The sufferer is turned, then, not to the "invisible things of God" but to the visible, suffering God in Jesus Christ.

Enlarging on this theme at book length, Walther von Loewenich discusses "life under the Cross." This theme is central to the Lutheran tradition: "The meaning of the cross does not disclose itself in contemplative thought but only in suffering experience." The real theologian makes discoveries not in the study or classroom but in the sickroom. He does not "shun suffering, but regards it as he would the holy relics, which are to be embraced devoutly." For God himself is "hidden in sufferings." If God's footprints are too visible in life, we have no need of faith. So faith more than works relates to suffering. The Christian life, says Loewenich, becomes "a discipline of suffering."

In this curious or paradoxical way of speaking Luther says that all objects of faith, if it is *really* faith, must be hidden. "It cannot, however, be more deeply hidden than under an object, perception, or experience which is contrary to it." So the all-powerful God is hidden in the weakness of Christ. All glory must be hidden in lowliness, nobility in disgrace, joy in grief, hope in despair, life in death. Christians must become like their Master in all things; his was, and theirs is to be a discipline of suffering. Christ's suffering is repeated in our lives. Suffering now is less important as a punishment for sin and more for the way it connects with faith. It becomes the surest way to God, a sign of God's grace, proof that we are God's children. Von Loewenich cites scores of Luther quotations to confirm these points.

The Christian life is "nothing else but following the cross." When Christians bear their cross they are doing nothing special, nothing that produces merits, but simply something that shows how believers and Christ are linked together.

> Therefore we must beware that the active life with its works and the contemplative life with its speculations do not lead us astray. Both are very attractive and peaceful, but for that reason also dangerous, until they are tempered by the cross and disturbed by adversaries. But the cross is the safest of all. Blessed is he who understands it.

All this means "being conformed to Christ." With this cross, then, can come peace, joy, happiness.[7]

The modern German Lutheran theologian Dietrich Bonhoeffer, who knew a life of affluence, comfort, and bourgeois success—only later to move under the cross and to death in a Nazi camp—carries the Lutheran tradition into a new age. In this period, the world is no longer naturally "religious." People no longer are moved by the power of God. They are stunned by or they ignore the divine weakness and silence. In such a setting Bonhoeffer pondered again the meaning of suffering. His is not the whole of the Lutheran tradition, but his restatement helps promote understandings for today, when so many of Luther's images are not culturally available.

One of many commentators who has picked up this theme in Bonhoeffer is André Dumas. We can judiciously follow his tracing of the suffering theme through Bonhoeffer. Bonhoeffer resurrected a word from the early church, the "secret discipline" by which the faithful lived in a culture that overwhelmed them. Today in a godforsaken age Christians should live by it again, so as not to parade false pieties and enthusiasms.

In light of this discipline, suffering comes to play a role Bonhoeffer called fellow believers to live: "the secret discipline of suffering." In 1934 he asked,

> Why is suffering holy? Because God suffers in the world through men. . . . Human suffering and weakness is a sharing in God's own suffering and weakness in the world. . . . Our God is a suffering God. Suffering forms man into the image of God. The suffering man is in the likeness of God.

Such suffering makes no claims of heroism, nobility, honor, or splendor—as it would necessarily in the case of Greek tragic heroes. Linked with Christ, this participation is instead simply an unavoidable reality.

At a crucial moment in his career, Bonhoeffer looked back and summarized not in the context of the sickroom, but appropriately for the ill as for all other suffering:

> It remains an experience of incomparable worth that we were able to look at the important events of world history from below—from the perspective of those who are left out, suspect, abused, powerless, oppressed, and mocked, in brief, those who are suffering. If only bitterness and envy have not corroded our hearts during this time, so that we may look upon stinginess and greatness, happiness and unhappiness, strength and weakness, with new eyes; that our vision of greatness and humaneness, of right and mercy, may have become clearer and less corruptible; that our personal

suffering may be a more suitable key, a more fruitful principle, a more contemplative and active opening to the world, than personal happiness would have been.

Such suffering permits resistance to evil. (Bonhoeffer was in the anti-Hitler underground.) It does not make believers passive in the face of illness. It also applies, however, to the world of pain, one that Bonhoeffer, even in prison, did not claim as his own. "I believe, for instance, that physical sufferings, actual pain and so on, are certainly to be classed as 'suffering.' We so like to stress spiritual suffering; and yet that is just what Christ is supposed to have taken from us...."

Suffering is not whimpering. "There is a kind of weakness that Christianity does not hold with," he said, in reaction against a complaining cellmate. Yet believers can show more measure of sympathy:

> We can share in other people's sufferings only in a very limited degree. We are not Christ, but if we want to be Christians, we must have some share in Christ's large-heartedness by acting with responsibility and in freedom when the hour of danger comes, and by showing a real sympathy that springs, not from fear, but from the liberating and redeeming love of Christ for all who suffer. Mere waiting and looking on is not Christian behavior.

Much of the discipline of Christian suffering, then, is supportive, sympathetic. It is the gathering or congregation sharing the burdens of the diseased or despairing in their midst. "Christians stand by God in his hour of grieving." That is "what distinguishes Christians from pagans." Bonhoeffer remembered Jesus asking, in Gethsemane, "Could you not watch with me one hour?"[8]

In the Lutheran witness to God, as Moltmann reminds us, "Christ and God form a unity not only in revelation, but already in their very being, as [Luther's] formula indicates: 'Christ alone and no other God.' Jesus Christ is 'the Lord Sabaoth.'" Moltmann quotes Luther further: "'The one whom the whole circle of the world never encompassed, lies in Mary's womb.'" In a Good Friday hymn, Johann Rist wrote:

> *O great distress, God himself lies dead,*
> *He died upon the cross,*
> *In this he won the kingdom of heaven*
> *For love of us.*

Later hymn books sometimes changed this to "God's son is dead," but before then radical theologians had spotted the birth of a "death-of-God theology" in Lutheran tradition.

In his nature God, of course, cannot die. But now that God and man are united in the one person, Jesus Christ, when the man dies, this is rightly called "the death of God, for he is one thing or one person with God."

Luther found ways to protect against the ancient heresy of "patripassianism," the idea that God the Father suffered in the death of Christ. We can set that issue aside for now. Here the point is that whatever else happens in Jesus Christ, this God comes to the point of being not powerful but weak, not glorious but suffering on the cross. Christians identify with that God in their suffering. God suffers alone and understands. Piety begins.[9]

Yet this "powerless" God, in other lights, does have the power to act. Therefore, the Christian may ask that the cup of suffering be taken away. The Lutheran tradition's view of suffering in the end does not lead one to wallow in weakness and gloom. There is, in the end, a triumphant note. "Our Lord God . . . did not make the head that I should hang it in this way; that is the way he created the beast." Although Luther soon stopped speaking about seeking suffering, he knew it would eventually find every believer. Werner Elert paraphrases him: "The night is terrible when God leaves us alone. But 'still it will come about that you are left alone.' Yet, 'trouble and anxiety . . . preserve us well in Christianity.'"

We would do an injustice to the Lutheran understanding of suffering if we left the victim in the dark night of the soul. There is a turnaround, for God was powerful to raise Christ, and God revisits the victim. "God shows His mastery [*Kunst*] by making something out of nothing, piety out of sin, life and holiness out of death." Christ is the real Conqueror of melancholy, since in his suffering he overcomes death. He commands us, "Rejoice, be happy, be confident; let not your heart be troubled," says Luther in his *Table Talk*. "Where Christ is, there joy is" (*Ubi Christus, ibi gaudium*).

> [Therefore] let everyone become a falcon, which can disappear on high in such trouble. Only let him first be certain, and let him not doubt, that God does not send him such trouble in order to destroy him . . . but that He wants to drive him to prayer, to calling, and to battle.

Luther's language is often this colorful: "If I want to be a Christian, I must also wear the court uniform, dear Christ does not supply any other garb at His court. *It is necessary to suffer.*"

Luther speaks of "the healing power of the holy cross." The time comes when Christians in faith turn their backs on the power of suffering. There is a time when God has to be concerned about the divine honor. "Just rout

suffering and the cross from your heart and mind to the best of your ability. Otherwise the evil becomes worse if you think about it for a long time."
Here Luther sounds like Dorothee Soelle in her blast against the "masochism of suffering."

In the long dark night of the hospital room the patient who identifies
with Christ experiences not only pain with which to struggle, but also a
puzzlement over the problem of pain. That same person does not use self-
help philosophy but, following the discipline of suffering, sees suffering to
the point where God acts again with the victory of faith.[10]

Part II

CARING
AND CURING

·4·
Caring:
Institutions, Roles, Practices

Whoever cares about health and medicine in the search for well-being is necessarily involved with the concept of care. Those who care treat a person in illness and greet a person in loneliness. One may be engaged in preventing illness and may be devoted to health foods, exercise, positive thinking, and general self-care. Still, the time comes when health fails. The sickroom door closes or the hospital room door opens. A victim becomes immobilized, dependent. Whether the disease is passing or permanent, a temporary setback or a terminal occasion, in times of need the one who is subject to that disease learns anew how important it is to be surrounded by individuals and agencies that are prepared to show care.

A WEAKNESS IN RESPECT TO JUSTICE

The Western religious traditions that derive from the Bible show such consistent concern for care that they hardly need depiction. It is a horror to suffer alone, to be relegated to the leper outpost or to the colonies of those who are shunned in their afflictions. It is a horror to be outside the circle of divine care. Any humans who close their hearts to the needs of others in illness come close to being put outside that circle, for God is love, and love issues in care.

Positively, to show care is one of the most affirmative ways to demonstrate the steadfast love of God who works through human beings. The widow, the orphan, and the sick become the tests of those moved by prophetic faith. In the New Testament, "inasmuch" as believers have cared for those in need, they have found Christ in the world and been Christs to their neighbors. Jesus may have engaged in extraordinary physical healing as a mark of his mission, but he also encouraged people to show ordinary care. The Good Samaritan parable is an excellent illustration of this test and evidence of love.

Within the larger Western traditions, specific heritages of church life have thier own specialities. The Lutheran tradition is not distinctive in that it finds some approaches to care more appropriate than others. To point to these is to indicate both the limits and the strengths of Lutheransim. After four and a half centuries we can judge that this heritage of Christianity has not been good at some works of care, whereas it has developed some reputation and finesse at others. Isolating the former can inspire reform. The Lutheran church claims to be open to constant re-formation. Pointing to the latter is not a basis for pride, but it is to outline a field in which there can be constant improvement.

To begin, then, with a broad generalization: Lutheranism has not excelled in and has rarely even entered the field of care that calls forth change in the structures and power relations of society. Complete care for others is based on moves for enacting justice, a justice that occurs on the scale of the nation, state, culture, society, or community. To do so one must work for reform through legislatures and policy-making agencies. The Calvinist tradition has developed far more heart and expertise in this respect than has the Lutheran. As H. Richard Niebuhr has shown, Calvinists believe, in broad lines, in the idea of "Christ Transforming Culture," in Christianizing the social order. This approach motivates them to work for change in the framework out of which care grows.[1]

Lutheranism, which has a more somber view of the way the demonic will continue to pervade existence until the end of history, has not found this similar motivation. It does not act as if its efforts in response to God will effect better structures, but calls instead for positive patterns of action in a world that will not be Christianized, in cultures that will not be transformed. This understanding has led to well-recognized charges that Lutheranism is politically passive, that it has missed the prophetic note that from ancient times down to today calls to judgment the oppressor, including the oppressor or those neglectful of the sick. The Lutheran tradition is more ready to work with the victims of a bad society than to change the society. In such work, it has patented its approaches to care and developed its specialties.

Retelling the Good Samaritan parable as it issues in policy is a good way of pointing to this distinction in approaches to care. Jesus in the gospel's retelling of the story speaks favorably of a Samaritan who did what Lutherans readily urge all people and especially all believers to do. He comes across a victim, someone who has through violence lost health, who is in need of medicine, and is far from being well. That Samaritan cares. He does not preach a sermon to save a soul and does not hand out tracts, but instead does what the situation demands. Wine and oil become his medicines, and a paid-up stay at the nearby inn is his equivalent of hospital care. All is well.

In the retelling, however, we are asked: would Jesus speak so positively if he had to report that the next day and the next and the next, ad infinitum, a poor man went down the road from Jerusalem to Jericho and was set upon by thieves and beat up? The Good Samaritan could have linked up with other people to improve the road, to assure better policing against highwaymen, to get at the roots of the problems that produced the thieves. In other words, through structural changes, he could have helped prevent the beatings in the first place. Would Jesus then congratulate the good but dumb Samaritan who daily made his way to pick up the pieces of a victim?

To point in such broad terms to specialties is not to suggest for a moment that Calvinism, for instance, has not developed good agencies, institutions, or impulses for care of the victims. Similarly, some Lutheran individuals, congregations, and movements have worked in Germany, Scandinavia, and America for social justice of a sort that effects good care. The two approaches are not clearly separated; the two styles are not chemically pure. Nor should one suggest that these styles are in competition; they can be complementary. Members of a congregation who begin acting by sending young people to sing Christmas carols in a senior citizens' home may soon involve themselves with the persons there. If they find that conditions in the home are bad because the state has poor licensing and regulating laws, they may be moved to lobby in the statehouse. Lutherans have been slower, however, to get on the bus for the trip to the capital than have members of many religious traditions.

In the third quarter of the twentieth century American churches, the Lutheran among them, experienced a form of awakening that led them to get at the political roots of oppressive and unjust measures. They worked for federal and state reform to include the rights of minorities to health care, to provide access by the poor to medical institutions that once had been denied them, or through Medicare and Medicaid to help assure some measure of dignity and security when it came to paying for care. The positive results of such programs were subjects of debate. Bureaucracies developed and, with them, some impersonality and carelessness came to be all too common.

In the beginning of the 1970s a reaction set in against bureaucracy, welfarism, and the like. A call from many came for a renewal in the private sector, a return for voluntary care to traditional institutions such as the family and church. It therefore may sound anachronistic to suggest that Lutheranism might better fulfill its mission by moving farther into the social welfare program at a time when others are having second thoughts. Yet if people attempt to gain some measure of objective distance on their political battles, they can recognize that intimate, personal, and congregationally based care of the ill and the suffering has to be connected with the larger political understandings in a complex industrial society. There will be reactions again to the reactions. Lutheranism is advised by many to care less about how to be relevant to a particular decade's political policies and more able to draw on the variety of Christian traditions in order to anticipate, head off, and treat problems that prevent well-being.

THE ARENA OF CARE

Without setting out to resolve that political issue, it is valid to concentrate on the half of the mandate and mission Lutheranism has readily accepted: immediate care. To document the notion that Lutherans have specialized in developing institutions of care or of providing congregations in which the ill are well treated would demand a writing of complex institutional history. Such a recounting is not the present point since this is not a book of information about all that Lutherans have or have not done. Instead, it points to what they believe their genius or character to be. What can we tell about a tradition of care that can be of help to people who want to be well, or to be of aid in helping others be well? Answers to that question determine the present plot.

The answers are very clear. First, as we have insisted from the beginning, Lutheran understandings grow out of their glowing core or center: the forgiveness of sins. Whatever Lutherans do by way of care is to be motivated by their understanding that bodily illness is connected with, a sign of, and an expression of a need that finds analogy in the necessity for forgiveness. The caring person therefore approaches the needy one in freedom, expressing a vocation that is called forth and sustained by the daily new start. The approach relies on an awareness of forgiveness.

The encounter with someone who is ill cannot be one of offering potions but of an announced word: "Your sins are forgiven." A followup on the part of the person with restored health is to live the forgiven life, to be an agent who embodies and transmits grace. The building of hospitals, wholistic care of the sick, and involvement of congregations and persons—all grow out of this experience of grace.

The other Lutheran distinctive has to do with "the universal priesthood of all believers." This is especially felt and displayed in the local congregation. Lutheran care has produced distinctive styles of pastorate. It has issued in the calling of the deaconess and the Christian nurse, doctor, or medical researcher—all of whom share equality before God in the church. They do not act as individuals but are expressive of the *Gemeinde*, the gathering or congregation. In turn, the gathering is a cell of the whole Christian Church.

Although a variety of callings has developed, Lutheranism finds "pastoral care," expressed through all of them, to display an urgent connection between the body of the faithful and a diseased person. Yet the body of the faithful as a whole is also summoned to be an agent of care.

The Lutheran chapters in books on "the cure of souls" are more prominent than would their corollary chapters be in books on "the care of bodies." In the Lutheran tradition, nevertheless, models for the second kind of books are to be drawn from the first kind. Books of the first sort concentrate on the two themes we have isolated. For example, John T. McNeill's standard-setting *History of the Cure of Souls* located a decisive moment in the story with the rise of the Lutheran Reformation. To be even more dramatic, "cure of souls," or the care of persons, was not to McNeill an effect of the Reformation, but a cause. McNeill opens his chapter: "In matters concerning the cure of souls the German Reformation had its inception." One does not write the history of Lutheranism and then see how care fits in. One writes a history of Christian care and sees how Lutheranism came out of it.

Martin Luther was both sick and sin sick. In seeking to satisfy his search for well-being he made demands that led to his invention of new (or restored) ways of care and cure. McNeill continues, "In Luther's theology [this first search] is to be associated with his doctrine of the common priesthood shared by all Christians, whereby we pray for others and share with them our spiritual gifts. Christ is where two or three are gathered in His name." There Christians "transmit the forgiven word and way of life to each other." All believers can use the Ten Commandments to "help to diagnose the soul's sickness." In treating sin, Luther viewed the subjects "with a pastoral eye rather than from the point of view of ecclesiastical authority."

McNeill's chapter provides instances that demonstrate the fusion between sin sickness and sickness in Luther's pastoral approach. At the supreme early crisis in his public life, as he prepared to appear at the Diet of Worms (where he issued his famed "Here I Stand!"), Luther took time to call on Hans von Minckwitz, a dying knight. "In the extreme pressure of his situation Luther might have secured for Minckwitz the services of another priest. But it was his habit to counsel the sick and dying." Also, "in 1527, during a visitation of the plague, he was faithful in attendance on the plague-stricken." Pastors, Luther insisted, "should no more take flight from pestilence than from a neighbor whose house is burning, or from one fallen into a pit."

Further:

> In Luther's Table Talk we have vivid stories that illustrate his ministry to the sick. "He conversed in a very friendly way" asking questions about the state of the sick man's body and soul. He commended to him Christian res-

olution and steadfast faith, and in reply to his expressions of gratitude explained that this was his office and duty. In bidding farewell he would remind the patient that God was a gracious Father, and that Christ had wrought our reconciliation. Amid such exhortations he counselled a man suffering from dropsy to do as his physicians ordered, that God's blessing might not be hindered by his anxiety. A woman showing violent symptoms of psychosis was led by his prayers to confess her sin of pride, and to pray for divine help, whereupon she was soothed to rest: after a relapse, she was ultimately cured.[2]

Such accents were not rare in Lutheranism. In a twentieth-century Library of Christian Classics one whole volume is devoted to *Luther: Letters of Spiritual Counsel.* The first chapter, over twenty-five pages long, is titled "Comfort for the Sick and Dying." The editor, without beginning to limit what Luther had to say, provides scores of examples. Other chapters deal with "Advice in time of Epidemic and Famine," intercessions for those in trouble or need, cheer for the anxious and despondent, and the like.

The editor's opening lines underscore McNeill's theme:

> Martin Luther (1483–1546) is usually thought of as a world-shaking figure who defied papacy and empire to introduce a reformation in the teaching, worship, organization, and life of the Church and to leave a lasting impression on Western civilization. It is sometimes forgotten that he was also—and above all else—a pastor and shepherd of souls.

For Luther and the tradition, counsel did not consist merely of applying external techniques but was "part and parcel of his theology." This was especially true as it related to sickness, which "played a large part in the lives of people in the sixteenth century." Luther, with the people of his day, might now and then passingly refer to sickness caused by sorcerers, but he usually saw illness to be natural, though in a sphere in which Satan still worked.

The writings of Luther make reference to care in respect to tuberculosis, ulcers, boils, abscesses, syphilis, scrofula, smallpox, inflammation of the eyes, fever, dysentery, epilepsy, apoplexy, jaundice, colic, dropsy, and stone. We mention them at this point to remind readers that to speak of spiritual care meant to be drawn into the very concrete world in which one who brings spiritual care deals with sanitation, diet, physicians, barbers, and apothecaries. Added to this is a focus that today would be called psychosomatic. "Our physical health depends in large measure on the thoughts of our minds. This is in accord with the saying, 'Good cheer is half the battle.'"

Care occurs in the context of the mass plague as well as individual illness. "Use medicine. Take whatever may be helpful to you. Fumigate your house, yard, and street. Avoid persons and places where you are not needed and where your neighbor has recovered. Act as one who would like to put out a general fire." Yet, advises Luther, do not run from the need for care. "Let everyone remain in his calling, for your neighbor needs your help and support. Do not forsake your neighbor." So Luther remained in Wittenberg in seasons of plague, visited the sick, and took some victims into his home. All this he connected with spiritual care.[3]

This notion that the Reformation itself was grounded in a pastoral care situation is confirmed in the later history of Protestantism and Lutheranism. Luther's model lives on in the tradition. Pastors are to be involved in care of the sick. They are called to represent the congregation at the side of the ill, to bring the sacraments to those who cannot be present in the gathering, in the name of the gathering. The pastor is not to run away from the plague and is to give highest priority to the sick. In any code of ethics for Lutheran pastors or in any assessing of strategic bases for ministry, the first call is to "drop everything" for the sake of calling on the sick. The lore of the pastorate is full of legendary, heroic attempts to interrupt what merely *seemed* important for the more important task of bringing spiritual counsel in illness. The lore of congregational distaste for bad pastors centers on their failure on this point. One may preach with the tongues of angels and still be dismissed if there is bedside neglect or if there are other signs of heartlessness. One is thought of as a good pastor, even though preaching is not eloquent, if the bedside manner is spiritually profound and caring.

In the 1970s American Lutherans undertook an intersynodical study of the "faces of ministry." This survey assessed the expectations of church members. The result took the form of a kind of message sent to the seminaries and parsonages. The authors wanted to make clear that congregational visions and agendas could not wholly determine the ministry. They knew that people who wish to be led often wish to be misled, as the writings of the biblical prophets already make clear. The surveyors regularly compared people's expectations with what they themselves thought priorities might be. Overall there was a consensus that people had grasped what ministry in the Lutheran tradition *ought* to be about. In the sample, 4033 lay persons gave their opinions in a body of 4,999, which included clergy.

The assumption behind our approach to traditions in ministry is confirmed in the survey. For all the friendliness shown all Christians in an ecumenical age, modern-day Lutheran congregants *did* want their pastors to reflect their tradition and lineage.

... Many Lutherans are unclear about what makes them distinguishable
from other Christians. But by asking a person what home life *should* be
like, one can often discover what that person's family life is like. When
one asks Lutherans what ministries they want, as we did, the hallmarks of
Lutheran-ness become visible in their replies.

Lutherans, the survey takers found, are identifiably Lutheran in their
insistence on the central theme of grace—"justification by faith." To this
they add a distinctive view of Christians as both sinners and saints. They
also emphasize that doctrine stands behind pastoral care in the first place.
"These emphases, though not unique to Lutherans, are nevertheless distinctive, highly valued, and well-nigh essential to the continuing identity
of Lutherans. If a pastor does not exhibit these distinctively Lutheran emphases, members of that congregation, even though unable to put their
fingers on exactly what is missing, will be uncomfortable."

The people emphatically did not want a doctrinal approach to be expressed legalistically or narrowly. They wanted it worked out in pastoral
care. Clergy even more emphatically than laity wished to measure themselves by this norm. "We discovered that Lutherans value pastors who (a)
are competent theologians, (b) are not dryly academic theologians, but
have integrated their theology into lives and beings, and (c) take a position
of critical acceptance of their Lutheran heritage—with about equal
emphasis on 'critical' and 'acceptance.'"

The real test of Lutheran distinctiveness was to be seen in how the pastor
was "a person for others." Members expect much by way of *diakonia*,
"serving the needs of people." Although this field rated sixth in a scale of
ten, it was ranked with administration and "community through Word
and Sacraments," and "contributes very much" to effective ministry. "Gracious availability" was a beautiful way of characterizing this. "And there
was my mother, dying in the hospital, and I called the pastor, and he
didn't even come!" This, says the authors, "in the eyes of many Lutherans,
would be a cardinal sin for any pastor to commit." Almost half of the sample (47 percent) considered it "absolutely essential" to an effective ministry
that a pastor "go immediately to minister to members in crisis situations."
However, "the issue is not only availability, but graciousness." There is to
be a calming influence in emergency situations, in nursing homes. There
must also be "empathetic aid in suffering."[4]

The quaint books devoted to preparing ministers some years ago reflect
the concern for well-being and in that respect are less dated than in most
others. Such books seem to anticipate every kind of human need from a
theological viewpoint. The most conservative of all, by John H. C. Fritz, is
characterized by sectarian narrowness. Fritz does not even ask for ecumen-

ical regard among Lutherans: the pastor "should accord non-Lutheran pastors, also pastors of other so-called [sic] Lutheran bodies, the common civilities demanded by good breeding and the law of Christian charity." That is all.

Such an author anticipates all forms of care in the light of his view of doctrine. We even get advice on baptizing two-headed babies as a dimension of pastoral care:

> Deformed children [*monstra, Missgeburten*] shall be baptized, provided they have a human head; for then it may be taken for granted that they have also a human soul. The opinion of the physician in such a case may be of value as also that of a brother clergyman. If deformed children have grown together and have two heads, it must be determined if there are *two individuals or only one.* If their bodies are mostly separate or grown together only at certain parts, and if each body shows independent action, as when one body sleeps while the other is awake or one laughs while the other cries, then it may safely be assumed that there are two distinct individuals with two distinct souls, and each individual therefore must be baptized.

Narrow, legalistic, and doctrinally obsessed though such a teacher of pastors may have been, even he did not underestimate the importance of well-being, both for the pastor who must be healthy to care, and then to care for health.

> *The Pastor's Health (physical fitness).* —To the spiritual and intellectual fitness of the pastor must be added physical fitness (I Tim. 5:23 [sic!]). A poor condition of health, a frail body, and a weakened constitution will greatly interfere with the work of a pastor. . . . He should therefore give attention to regular habits of life, to diet, sleep, exercise, and recreation. . . .

> Next to regular habits of living, health and strength can best be preserved, and also be best acquired, by fresh air (open windows by day and night, outdoor life, deep breathing), wholesome food (all kinds, a variety, vegetables, not too much meat, food well prepared, no overeating, drinking much water, a well-balanced diet), sufficient amount of sleep . . . and bodily exercise (taken daily in the open air, —walking is best exercise, —calisthenics, gardening, etc.).

Given such a background, we are not surprised to see that "the cure of souls" accents pastoral calling for bodily and health care through visiting the sick. Sick calls are often taken for granted: "The making of pastoral calls should not be limited to visiting the sick . . . " (although these should be given first consideration). Again, "it is a most solemn duty of every pastor to visit the sick and the dying . . . . " In Luther's spirit, "a contagious or infectious disease or some disgusting malady should never keep a Christian pastor away from the bedside." Fritz refers to a tract by Luther for warrant. He provides lengthy counsel on how to avoid being infected. He also depicts some division of labor: "The physician seeks to alleviate and cure the bodily disease, pain, and distress, but the greater, mental and spiritual, agony and distress can be relieved and cured only by words of divine consolation."

Reading such an archaic volume for specific counsel today would be beside the point. The art of pastoral care has been greatly improved in the fifty years since Fritz wrote. What is important is to see how he picked up the central Lutheran theme. Pastoral care involves cheer: the announcement of grace, word, voice, speaking, addressing, praying, conversing, communing, are the accents of his pages. "Many an ill is due to a wrong mental or spiritual attitude, and therefore the resulting unhappiness and even bodily discomfort are self-inflicted and avoidable. The Christian religion is a happy and cheerful religion," so the cure has to come from a heart moved by the words of grace and cheer.[5]

An earlier volume in the American tradition, G. H. Gerberding's *The Lutheran Pastor*, seems less quaint in some of its counsel and bears at least as clearly the main themes of the Lutheran tradition in pastoral care. Like Fritz, Gerberding more than most Lutherans later in the century, accents the "chastening" and personal aspect of illness by a punishing God. He then quotes Augustine to the effect that pastors who neglect to visit the sick are *desolators* instead of *consolators*. "The pastor . . . comes to the sick-bed as the minister of the Word. . . . The pastor is not to play the physician or to interfere with him." But he can aid "by giving a few hygienic directions" and by counseling congregants how to visit the sick. "We have come in contact with many unbelieving physicians. But when they understand our ways and ideas, they never once objected to our methods."[6]

Most of the more sophisticated recent literature on pastoral care, from the pioneering work of Granger Westberg, William E. Hulme, and David Belgum to the countless experts on clinical pastoral education, is more ecumenical and open to secular counsel. Yet all the authors reflect these central Lutheran themes of care: its priority and urgency; its representation of the believing community; its base in Word and Sacrament; its central focus on "cheer" in the word of grace; the need for understanding sickness in connection with sin sickness; the importance of teamwork with physicians and other medical personnel.

THE ROLE OF COMMUNITY

It may seem strange to spend so much energy on pastoral care in a chapter devoted to the Lutheran accent on "the universal priesthood of all believers." The pastor, however, is somehow a representative person in the congregating link. Yet most care must be undertaken by lay people, who greatly outnumber pastors, spend more time with the sick, and have to be equipped to carry out the works of mercy.

Some Lutheran counselors, for example the pioneering Granger Westburg, have spent much energy equipping people in healing professions to carry their Christian care into the sickroom. Thus Westberg wrote *Nurse, Pastor, and Patient,* arising from his Lutheran-Protestant viewpoint, but for all Christians. His accent is on nurses' faithfulness in vocation, opportunities for special kinds of care, and circumscribed occasions for use of the healing Word to go with medicine and healing hand. These chapters are typical of the aspects of care that are most congenial in the Lutheran tradition.[7]

Here the concept of vocation is urgent in matters of care. Non-Lutheran writers on this theme of care, which honors the role of nurse, physician, and lay person, also cite Luther. Thus Baptist Wayne Oates lifts up the theme of "the priesthood of all believers . . . in that it affirms the duty of all Christians to serve one another in love in all stations of life." Morale building by Christians in this field is a prime task:

> The psychologist, the psychiatrist, the social worker, the penologist, the internal medicine expert—can from their stations in life sustain a Christian in his distress. In turn, the Christian has a ministry to render to them. They too have need of a friend, a confidant, a pastor, a shepherd. They are not sufficient unto themselves. . . . If, by the grace of Christ, they should become Christians, they would still function as always in their stations in life. Martin Luther . . . says of the shepherds that they went to see the child Jesus: "The Scripture says plainly that they returned and did exactly the same work as before. They did not despise their service, but took it up again where they left off with all fidelity, and I tell you that no bishop on earth ever had so fine a crook as those shepherds."[8]

The lay people who exercise the priesthood of all believers may, in an emergency, baptize; ordinarily they participate in Holy Communion under pastoral care, but there has also been a trend in modern Lutheranism to set aside, call, and equip deacons to take the sacrament to the sick. This practice developed not just as a pastoral time-saver or a substitute for pastoral care, but it is another sign of care by the congregation. Lay ministry is to bear most of the same marks as the pastoral in respect to

Christian care. Yet the laity has also been called upon to generate agencies
and systems of care for the physical needs of people. Here Lutheranism
likes to see its heritage to be rich and long.

From a shelf full of possibilities, a sample is Richard W. Solberg's *As Between Brothers: The Story of Lutheran Response to World Need.* Solberg
tells the story of care in the form of world relief. He shows quite plausibly
that modern Lutherans found each other across synodical lines and organized themselves as a confession through the Lutheran World Federation
and national agencies for the purpose of care. World War I and World
War II were the great impetuses. "When this period of sharing began, the
Lutheran churches of the world knew very little about one another." The
priesthood of believers was deepened through "a community of suffering"
and a "fellowship in blessing."[9]

Since we are making much of "the priesthood of all believers" as a Reformation theme of Lutheran patent and a key to the tradition of care, we advisedly lift it up for closer view. The theme does not represent simply
"democracy in the church," "the right of private judgment," or "individualism, independent of the clergy." These are all later, accidental, or
alien corollaries of the original notion. Cyril Eastwood, in tracing the concept from the Reformation to the present day, sees the roots of the tradition
in Luther himself. We shall, with Eastwood, revisit a few of the themes
that have most bearing on this tradition's approach to care.

The notion begins in the preaching of the Word of God. Luther said,
"The soul can do without everything except the Word of God." His *Large
Catechism* makes clear that unlike the Episcopal church, where the ministry is placed above the church, for Lutheranism "the Ministry is placed in
the congregation." The congregation assures the concrete character of the
Word. "When I have called the Church a spiritual assembly, you have in-
sultingly taken me to mean that I would build a church as Plato builds a
state that never was." A Platonic idea does not care for people. A modern
Lutheran, K. E. Skydsgaard, accents this: "The predominating concept is
that of the Congregation or People.... Here the chief stress falls. It is
therefore consistent with this that our Churches attach great significance
to the priesthood of all believers; and the practical consequence of this is
that the laity play a very real part in our Church life."

In the Lutheran tradition, "priesthood and laity" are in unity; they
share a common dignity. Baptism consecrates all without exception "and
makes us all priests," says Luther. Here is a charter for medical professionals and Christians who care for the sick as amateurs:

A shoemaker, a smith, a farmer, each has his manual occupation and
work; and yet, at the same time, all are eligible to act as priests and bish-

ops. Every one of them in his occupation or handicraft ought to be useful
to his fellows, and serve them in such a way that the various trades are all
directed to the best advantage of the community, and promote the well-
being of body and soul, just as the organs of the body serve each other.

All Christians therefore are called to serve. They share a common privilege
in this. They act to channel forgiveness in the world of need.

The final test of the sufficiency of faith in a Christian is the service of her
neighbor. As Luther said,

All that we do must be designed for the benefit of our neighbour, because
each one has sufficient for himself in Christ. [The Christian] should have
no other thought than of what is needful to others. That would mean living a true Christian life; and that is the way in which faith proceeds to
work with joy and love.... To my neighbour, I will be, as a Christian,
what Christ has become to me.[10]

The interplay of the ordained and the laity displays the spread of Lutheran agencies of mercy designed to help promote well-being. Annual
volumes of the *Lutheran Health and Welfare Directory* canvass these
agencies and suggest something of the scope of involvement. A code at the
beginning of the volume points to the variety of services: six types for "services to the aging"; thirteen for "child welfare"; five for "family welfare";
three for "health services," including "general" and "special" hospital and
"mental health clinic"; four services to handicapped adults; and many
kinds of settlement and resettlement agencies. These codes connect with
hundreds of identified institutions in North America. Those institutions do
not begin to suggest the dimensions of care in modern Lutheranism. Congregations also may generate their own.[11]

The shift from early, simpler, Lutheran congregational and individual
care to the more complex forms resulted from the changes brought by the
industrial revolution in the last two centuries. These transformed the tradition and called for the new institutions and approaches. The story of
some of these appears in William O. Shanahan's *German Protestants Face
the Social Question*, a pioneering effort at seeing the Lutheran (and other
Reformation) traditions change in the face of societal pressure.

Shanahan's book is still the best place to learn what a conservative tradition could or could not do in a time of upheaval. He speaks of "the *evangel-
ical-social movement*" in Germany in the nineteenth-century churches of
the Reformation heartland. This movement combined the idealism of contemporary Germany with "Luther's sober estimate of man's powers to deal
with the natural world." Before then, "by proposing to deal only with individual cases of need, charity generally overlooked the social causes of
human misery. Nor did charity promise remedial action."

Shanahan develops a history of the social ethic on German Lutheran soil, a subject that awaits further development. For now, the important theme to trace is the rise of "new charities and new orthodoxy," in the nineteenth century. A new Pietism combined with a kind of romantic doctrinal recovery—together they were called the Awakening. Lay people expressed "the universal priesthood of believers." As in England and the United States, agencies for tract dissemination and missionary activity developed. A burst of activity to aid children who were victims of industrial change marked the movement.

The new concept of care involved women as never before. Thus Theodor Fliedner helped devise an order of deaconesses. He resurrected a biblical name for their office in order to minimize opposition to it. The title was officially authorized in Prussia in 1844. These women who took on ascetic roles comparable to those of Catholic nuns, spread the work of care in deaconesses' houses and hospitals.

The giant in the field of care during the nineteenth century was Johann Hinrich Wichern (1808–81), an expert diagnostician of the age's ills, a practical reformer and builder of institutions. A conservative enemy of the legacy of the French Revolution, Wichern worked within the context of conservative social policy to improve the circumstances of those who needed care. He saw prostitutes, thieves, and delinquents ruining youths and despoiling cities. "Fundamentally, Wichern remained a Lutheran particularly in recognizing that salvation lies in faith. It was his genius to see that the creativity of faith also had a worldly meaning."

In 1833 Wichern, on the property of his patron near Hamburg, invented a *Rauhes Haus* or an "unkempt place" for the young. It became the chief agency of social enterprise in Lutheran Germany. There Lutheran styles of care blended with the new German idealism, as it became a model for diaconal work. At the center of this activity, says Shanahan, Wichern placed the "Lutheran doctrine of the priesthood of all believers." People in the *Rauhes Haus* served each other while they were being served.

No new movement can express "the Lutheran tradition" unequivocally or without hazard of opposition. As Wichern's "Inner Mission" developed, the conservative Lutheran churches of Mecklenburg, Hanover, and Saxony opposed it, however timid it may have been. "Their leaders feared that the lay resources mobilized in voluntary associations would make the Inner Mission a 'church within a church.'" Wichern was therefore always on the defensive. Yet he picked up friends in the theological faculty at Erlangen and eventually won a way for it. Wichern's strength lay in his typical Lutheran belief that if he concentrated on declaring the Word of God to the sick and the poor, they would themselves become renewing agents. At last and at least, he convinced Lutheranism's conservative side of the understanding that "material circumstances have a bearing upon man's spiritual life."

As Wichern broadened his program, he lost support; but an important ally remained in Wilhelm Löhe (1808–72), a great missioner, healer, institution builder, and link between European and American Lutheranism. He founded a settlement at Neuendettelsau to care for the physical needs of people in the context of Lutheran sacramentalism. The impetus soon crossed the ocean. Among the heroes and heroines of American Lutheranism are such hospital builders as William Passavant (1821–94). Passavant, a Pennsylvanian, helped import deaconess work into America and founded hospitals in Chicago, Milwaukee, and Pittsburgh, and orphanages in several cities.

To trace the history of hospital building is not our purpose; the Lutheran form differs too little from that of other evangelical denominations. However, it is important to see this particular form of "the priesthood of all believers" as a ministry that combined cure and care. Lutherans feel at home with it and see it as their main more-than-congregational contribution to human well-being. From that center other Lutheran understandings grow. The area of ethics and justice has meanwhile remained a greater problem in respect to the Lutheran tradition in medicine and care.[12]

·5·

Healing: The Acts of Healing, the Arts of Prayer

From the beginning and through most places and times, the Lutheran tradition has connected healing with both spiritual and medical resources. Not even the modern Lutheran charismatic movement—linked with Pentecostalism and thus at least potentially suspicious of science—calls its adherents to repudiate the work of researchers, clinicians, surgeons, or pharmacists. At the same time, this tradition has always regarded healing as belonging to the special care of God. It has consistently advocated petitionary and intercessory prayer for healing. This means asking for one's own well-being and loving the neighbor on one's knees.

That Lutherans believe in medicine and prayer alike seems unremarkable. Awareness of this belief hardly looks like aid today for people who seek well-being. Yet often when people reexplore what they have always taken for granted it becomes evident that there were few reasons to have taken it for granted. What seems to be a natural coming together was originally the result of serendipity, accident, mutations, or unexpected foresight.

THE RISE OF "SECULAR" SCIENTIFIC MEDICINE

Should modern-day inheritors of the Lutheran tradition take for granted its consistent embrace of science and medicine? Whenever a Lutheran Christian takes ill, the congregation at once calls upon the resources of the hospital and clinics. Why should this be? Are not some of the assumptions of science in conflict with the concepts of healing in the gospels, concepts that Lutherans regularly revisit and celebrate? Some Lutherans are suspicious of some other aspects of science. There have been strong strands of antievolutionary attitudes in conservative Lutheranism. Many modern technological discoveries were first greeted as threats to faith. "Science versus faith" has been a popular topic in many a Lutheran campus discussion in America. College students often question this relationship because they were taught to feel a strain between science and faith.

Lutheranism developed at a moment in Western history when the language of science was taking a new turn. There were reasons for its leaders to react against the rise of this science, which so often seemed to be displacing both God and humankind from the center of the universe. The church, being traditional, sometimes reacted instinctively against the new. It mistrusted the unfamiliar. For that reason, the new discoveries in medical science could have come as a threat, and on occasion they were.

German theologian Gerhard Ebeling somewhere noted that during the Protestant and Catholic Reformation the leading thinkers fought over the inherited scholastic "ation" words, such as *expiation, propitiation,* and *justification.* These terms could fossilize once-living concepts of how God deals with humans. By the sixteenth century some of these concepts were passé and appeared dated in the textbooks. Meanwhile, as Catholic and Protestant picked over dead bones and cared for antique shops, the new world of science—the world of Copernicus, Tycho Brahe, Johannes Kepler, and Paracelsus—was breaking open around the Christian thinkers. People were looking to new sources for explanations. A change in explanations is an assault on understandings, understandings that in the present case had been with the church for centuries.

Through the modern centuries, however, much of the impetus for the hospital and medical research has come on the largely Lutheran soil of northern Europe in Scandinavia and especially in Germany. The German university, laboratory, and hospital for some time was the world-renowned arena for advanced medicine. Some of the scientists and physicians ignored the faith of their foreparents and let it play no part in their present thinking. Others opposed this faith. But the biographies of these figures show that many remained faithful church members who seldom heard anything from the pulpit to upset their scientific thinking.

Some theologians have asked whether special resources reside in the faith itself to make possible the impulse toward scientific inquiry. Critics of the Christian momentum like to argue that the first chapter of the first book of the Bible, which says that humans should "have domain over creation" (Gen. 1:28), has led them to seek mastery, to dominate. Nature demands response. It suffers or fights back when humans use its resources too rapidly and unthinkingly. In this reading, from Genesis on, the biblical story and those who later accept it conspire to impel people to violate nature, to lose spiritual resources in the natural order.

German Lutheran theologian Friedrich Gogarten made much of this "secularizing" aspect of biblical and Protestant, especially Lutheran, thought. This form of faith believes in the Lordship of Christ. Everything that goes on in the universe, the created order, and especially the human world operates somehow under the creating, provident, and caring hand of God. That being the case, there is no reason for the Christian to have to pounce nervously on all human endeavor and name it "anonymously" Christian. There has been among Lutherans little talk about Christianizing the social order or transforming the world of politics, arts, science, and letters. In Lutheran eyes, the demonic keeps on pervading the orders of existence. It does not, it will not, go away in history. The world is not progressively turning into the Kingdom of God. One does not wait for it to do so.

In a phrase of Swedish Bishop Gustaf Aulén, Lutherans, when true to their own tradition, recognize that it is necessary "to let everything be what it is." There is no expectation that every good work in medicine must occur at a Christian hospital. Researchers into things of the body do not have to feel that the body is the Temple of the Holy Spirit in order to be effective. No, they say, let the secular be the secular. The scientist or physician may let the world round itself off without reference to divine symbols, to God's saving activity.

Of course, Lutherans express a strong hope that researchers or medics will be found by the grace of God, for the sake of their souls. There is also an understanding that a spiritual view of the body will motivate reliable care and carefulness. But the gifts of healing come not only to or through the Christian or through the Lutheran churchgoing doctor. The Lord of history is active in the Jewish hospital and in the public clinic, where no Christian symbols of any sort beckon or define. Let medicine be medicine, whatever else it becomes.

The Lutheran tradition equally "lets God be God," as Philip Watson summarized the Lutheran theology. Letting God be God means that the believer does not claim to have a monopoly on divine explanations, to know what is going on in the sacred majesty. For that reason, there is less recourse here than in some other traditions to the notion of a separate supernatural sphere to which the believer seeks access through the use of anointing oils, the laying on of hands, or special prayers of healing designed to induce miracles.

One modern scholar proposes that Christians speak of the "ordinary" and "unusual" instead of "natural" and "supernatural." Wade H. Boggs, Jr., proposed to abandon the very distinction between "natural" and "supernatural," especially as these apply to healing.

> . . . the truth of the matter is that Martin Luther rejected this Catholic distinction at the beginning of the Protestant Reformation. A group of the best scholars in the English free churches, at the request of the Archbishop of Canterbury, have recently summarized the essentials of Luther's theology. With reference to Luther's views about nature, they say, "So

far, then, from developing and extending the medieval antithesis between nature and grace, *Luther repudiates it entirely. . . .*" [Luther] thereby precluded any possibility of an independent, self-administering nature, and made unnecessary and meaningless the idea of God "intervening" in His own world. As extraordinary or emergency situations arise, God can and no doubt will continue to act in new and different ways. We may even be surprised by some of these divine procedures with which we may be as yet unfamiliar, and refer to them as miracles. But even so, we have no right to label them "supernatural," because they are just as "natural" to God as are His habitual acts.[1]

Not all scholars, not all Lutherans, would insist on such a surgically severe abolition of the "natural/supernatural" distinction. There are ways in which it can be brought into play. The modern Lutheran charismatic movement is trying to keep it alive or to restore it in reformed ways. What Boggs refers to, as the reasons for doing *something* about the medieval distinction, however, does come close to the heart of the Lutheran tradition. Its adherents believe in healing, in being healed, in drawing on the resources of faith for healing. At the same time, they show some measure of mistrust when they hear extravagant claims for "supernatural intervention." At the very least, believers are taught to be careful about claiming that they know the details of such intervention. Too direct applications of the language of intervening miracle set people up for an eventual crisis of faith and loss of trust when there is no subsequent "intervention." Is God then capricious, playing games with the ill?

To this point I have simply been trying to insist that the Lutheran tradition, while fully moved by faith in the divine power of God the healer, is also matter of fact and realistic. It celebrates the ordinary means of healing—as if one can speak of modern medical discoveries as ordinary. It never stops relying on the unusual that results from Christian people coming to act in faith and trust in the divine Savior and Healer. Wherever there is a strong push for teaching a mistrust of the power of medicine or the power of God, one becomes aware that there is also a straying to the edges of or beyond the borders of the Lutheran tradition.

THE CONCEPTS OF VOCATION AND INTERCESSION

One point at which the tradition weds what in some traditions are divorced is in the concept of the vocation. The vocation means the calling, the call, the understanding of how the forgiven sinner each day is liberated to act. The power of God that comes with each sun's rising sets believers loose to pursue honest professions and patterns of work, to accept what each day brings by way of opportunity or threat.

The believer who is a nurse does what God calls him to do through the daily rounds of the wards. The Christian who is doctor responds in faith to the challenges of her clinic, not always having to pause and "religiocify," supernaturalize, or slow things down by rendering into pious language what the day demands. The one who prays, the representative of a congregation, the minister who brings communion to the sick and the visitor —all also live in a vocation. Through it they see divine power in the ordinary and recognize their own assigned roles in healing.

Such an approach locates healing in both the hospital and the prayer chamber. Prayers of petition and intercession are a major part of all Lutheran approaches to healing. Each week tens of thousands of congregations lift up the names of those who are ill, who are in physical need. They intercede not merely as a courtesy, a sign of club life. They also do not thus pray in the hope that God will always intervene with miracles from a supernatural order. Lutherans pray that they will come to understand God's actions in the lives of the bed-ridden and dying. They hope that God will give comfort and healing to those in need. Prayer changes the pray-ers. Prayer changes things.

So much does the concept of the interceding congregation play a part in thoughts about healing that Luther developed the biblical concept of a "priesthood of all believers" to include the concept and its practice. To some, this "priesthood" has meant simply a democratization of clerical roles. In that case, all are seen as doing the work of the ordained or the professional cleric. Not at all. Numbers of scholars have pointed out that the priesthood of all believers was a concept that stressed how all believers could approach God, as priests alone once did, thus representing the community in intercessory prayer.

The Lutheran tradition may reject some "natural versus supernatural intervention" thinking, but part of it also stands in the biblical lineage. More is there described by way of prayerful healing than our picture of Lutheranism at this point portrays. Thus, on many occasions in the New Testament, Jesus does *not* work signs or engage in healing. At other times he does participate by calling forth faith and prayer. In some instances there *are* healing miracles. In the early church special means were often taken to connect the would-be healed with the Healer. What does Lutheranism do about these?

THE PRAYER OF HEALING

The charismatic Lutheran, who, as a noncharismatic church leader once put it to me, "comes easily within the allowable spectrum," would say that the tradition has allowed New Testament healing forms to atrophy. Lutheranism has the option to retrace its steps, forget about the magic it was fighting off in sixteenth-century Catholicism, and turn to New Testament practices. In a day when so many discoveries in science and faith occur, we would be ill-advised to hurry past this set of options. Its long-latent resources contain a possibility for promoting well-being; the inquirer within the Lutheran tradition advisedly engages in *ressourcement,* which means going deeper into the tradition. If Luther represented rediscovery in the church, then those in his tradition should be open to new stirrings of the Spirit and go behind him.

The charismatic movement, details of which we need not pursue here, is a descendant of the Pentecostalism that broke forth in American Protestantism at the turn of the century. Revivalists in the Pentecostal-Holiness tradition around 1900 in Kansas, 1906 in Los Angeles, and then in many times and places, experienced startling phenomena. They began to sing or speak in tongues, *glossolalia,* a form of unrepressed, unintelligible speech. The New Testament pictures this as one of the lesser but allowable spiritual gifts. To the Pentecostalists this visitation by the Holy Spirit signaled a new age. With it came the gift of interpretation. Pentecostalists, on the basis of some New Testament traces, soon began to speak of a "second baptism," a "baptism of the Holy Spirit," without water, a seal of conversion. From the beginning, such Pentecostal people included the New Testament gifts of healing among the Spirit's blessings.

Although these forms of Pentecostalism were largely dismissed in mainline churches as "holy roller," "snake handling," and the like, out of it grew a new phenomenon. It took rise in middle-class denominations between 1960 and 1966—in Lutheranism around 1961–63. This type of Pentecostalism tends to choose the word *charismatic* to describe itself, both to distinguish itself from the older "sectarian" forms and to stress the "gifts of the spirit." Such Episcopalians, Roman Catholics, and Lutherans have not been content merely to be charismatics but want to find roots in their own traditions, since only their extremists have been eager to move out of the existing churches. These charismatics have had to recognize that the more vivid and even spectacular "charismatic gifts" were not part of the regular practice in their traditions. Most of the earlier articulators of these traditions acted as if, or even said, that the gifts of tongues, healing, prophecy, and interpretation had belonged distinctively to the first Christian generation.

Lutheranism from the beginning showed a genuine distrust of the claim that these gifts were again present in a later day. Luther almost lost his own sense of well-being whenever he had to deal with what he called "enthusiasts." These were people who claimed identification with or a possession of—or a being possessed by—the Spirit. Remembering the biblical picture of the Holy Spirit as a dove, Luther once accused a spiritist, "You swallowed the Holy Ghost, feathers and all." Revelation came only through the Word of God, Jesus Christ, as witnessed to in the Holy Scriptures. So Lutherans mistrusted anyone who claimed that the Holy Spirit talked to or through them directly. The world around early Lutheranism was so shot full of magic and superstition that the founders showed a horror of turning to modes of healing that might encourage any too ready recourse to a sense of magic-plus-miracle. Perhaps the reaction was too extreme.

The Lutheran charismatic who seeks an anchor in tradition or a set of precedents does not have much to go on in the career of Luther. A single incident, however, stood out. One reads about it almost ad nauseam in the histories of Christian healing or the charismatic literature. Clearly, it shows that Luther had some faith in "faith healing." Yet by its rareness and vagueness it also succeeds in showing that first-generation Lutheranism showed little interest in "special means."

After Martin Luther counseled Prince Philip of Hesse to practice bigamy and then to lie about the situation, his conscientious colleague Philip Melanchthon, seeing himself as a coconspirator, felt guilty. Melanchthon fell deathly ill. Luther discovered his fellow reformer in a near-comatose state. He looked at Melanchthon fondly, deliberately, with concern. Then he retired to a window corner and prayed. As the story goes, after prayer Luther grasped his colleague's hand and said, "Be of good courage, Philip, you will not die; give no place to the spirit of sorrow, and be not your own murderer, but trust in the Lord, who can stay and make alive again, can wound and bind up, can smite and heal again."[2] Melanchthon, in this pious story, subsequently recovered his health. Charismatics called this "a therapeutic miracle."

Admittedly, this is not much to go on. It pales when contrasted with the televised Pentecostal evangelists and their claimed healings. Yet the incident, marginal though it may seem, shows that Luther could be deliberate about calling upon "special prayers of healing" in special circumstances. One dare not make much of it, but neither should one make nothing at all of it.

Scholastic orthodoxy was militant against claims of special gifts of the spirit, but Lutheranism produced Pietist movements in which both congregational intercessory prayer and visiting the sick were warmly practiced. Still, one cannot speak of the gift of healing as having been pursued in most Lutheran circumstances through the centuries. There have been exceptions. The most notable was a "charismatic" or spirit-filled teacher and pastor, Johan Christoph Blumhardt (1805–1880) of Germany. Indeed, we may speak of him as the founder of modern Lutheran healing movements.

In his small-town congregation, two sisters, Katherina and Gottliebin Dittus, seemed possessed by poltergeists. For two years their pastor prayed over them, yet one sister only became more disturbed, more convulsive. One night as she was restrained in a chair she heard that Satan was claiming power over her and that Christ alone could triumph. Finally, as Blumhardt prayed the woman shouted, *"Jesus ist Sieger,"* Jesus is Victor. By morning she was healed. She later worked with Blumhardt.

Given the long history of Christian exorcism, the story is unremarkable. Something like that must have gone on tens of thousands of nights throughout Lutheran history. Yet this one took on legendary character because Blumhardt went on to found a movement. The cure issued in a religious revival in 1845, at which Blumhardt practiced the laying on of hands. People were healed, or considered themselves to be healed. Blumhardt's ministry outgrew his parsonage. In 1852 he established a Christian healing center at Bad Boll, a sulphur springs spa.

Blumhardt revealed the degree of his repose in the Lutheran tradition by remaining close to the medical profession and encouraging that the ill accept its ministrations. He also played down any notions of the supernatural or superstition. He was dealing at the borderline where faith turned the ordinary into the unusual. Blumhardt was opposed to the idea that prayer was a contest of wills in which God is induced to heal. It is not something God otherwise would not have done. The German healer was ready with explanations or he had the faith to be content with the absence of explanations, whenever healing did not come. His was a call to a new way of life, of fresh openness to the ways of God. Blumhardt, who combined this charismatic healing with a social ministry, is revered as someone who opened a new page in Lutheran understandings of healing.

The contemporary charismatic movement, that allowable option in one zone of Lutheranism, picks up on the Melanchthonism incident, the Blumhardt example, and a few other moments in Lutheran history. Then it asks for a return to the New Testament and borrows from non-Lutheran history in order to make a new set of claims or offer prescriptions. In a few rare congregations the Lutheran charismatics have departed from their tradition and scorned medical help, but the leadership has always tried responsibly to keep the old alliances alive.

A typical contemporary advocate is Pastor Larry Christenson, whose *The Charismatic Renewal Among Lutherans* includes a chapter on healing. Significantly, he rests his whole case on the Bible, never on the

Lutheran tradition. Christenson recalls the times in which Saint Paul, so revered in the tradition, healed. At Lystra Paul's command to a cripple from birth, "Stand up on your feet" (Acts 14:10), resulted in a healing. In Ephesus people carried to the sick some handkerchiefs or aprons that Paul had touched. The diseases left them (Acts 19:11–12). Christenson says of this, "Paul put them in touch with the healing power of God." Paul healed the father of a leading citizen on Malta (Acts 28:8–9). Paul, writes this modern pastor, was not content merely to preach the gospel in human wisdom and eloquence; he spoke with power. Then Christenson intrudes to scold the noncharismatics of his own time:

> Much present-day preaching of the gospel is exactly reversed. We hold no fear of preaching the gospel with a brilliant display of human wisdom and eloquence: Flawless progression of logic and rhetoric, replete with histor- ical and literary allusions, psychologically persuasive, intellectually re- spectable, philosophically palatable, appealing to one's sense of morality and responsibility, emotionally uplifting. This kind of preaching can go on week after week, month after month, year after year—faultless in form and even thoroughly orthodox in doctrine—yet with no manifesta- tion of God's power whatever. Do we *fear* this kind of preaching, as Paul did? We don't. We admire it. Laymen stand in awe, and preachers in envy. But let the *power* of God so much as be mentioned—prayers for healing, anointing with oil, exorcism, the demonstration of the Spirit— just mention this, and people draw back in fear and doubt.

Christenson's defensiveness shows that he knows he is invoking corners of his church's tradition against larger numbers who claim its center. He resents it when others see means as being frills or options. No, Paul would have insisted they were integral to the faith.

Christenson proceeds: *"Is healing according to the will of God?"* Every Lutheran would answer yes, but Christenson here means healing through the instruments that the charismatic movement favors. Yes, Jesus carried on an active ministry of healing. The healing ministry of the church follows from belief in the indwelling Christ. "There is no word in Scripture which suggests that healing would outdo its usefulness in the church or in glorifying God. Jesus . . . has never said, 'I do not desire to heal any longer.'" People, by using only human reason, came toward *that* conclusion. Christenson cites a Presbyterian report and an Episcopal cleric, not Lutheran tradi- tion, to reinforce his themes.

Healing in all these ways "was never meant to be an option" for "those who like to go off on special talents." Instead, those who shun it fail to preach the whole gospel. Christenson complains that people object: "Oh, it can lead to fanaticism! People might lose their faith if you pray for some-

one and then he dies! We have modern medicine now and don't need healing by prayer! Faith healers are all quacks anyway!" There *are* dangers in
the movement, he admits; there has been abuse. But "the *neglect* of the
ministry of healing has a danger that outweighs them all: *the danger of dis-
obeying the Lord.*" The church now lacks obedience. Christenson feels
that the Lutheran charismatic movement is sufficiently disciplined. It cautions against weird emotionalism or worldly supernaturalistic claims. He
quotes Lutheran Karlfried Froehlich in a passage that applies to healing:

> Could the charismatic phenomena of our day be seen as manifestations of
> the Spirit in a new, concrete human form? Could the yearning of Chris-
> tians for the experience of charismatic phenomena be understood as part
> of that incarnational emphasis, the longing for something concrete, real,
> down-to-earth to express what has been there in a lofty way already?
>
> Could it be that Martin Luther himself would side with the charismatic
> movement in the church today for precisely the same reasons that forced
> him to reject what he saw as the flight from this earth in the Enthusiasts
> [the people who too readily claimed the Spirit in Luther's day]?

Lutheran charismatics such as Christenson are not eager to disrupt their
churches. They are scrambling for elements of the tradition that will ground
their movement, and they counsel adaptation. He is explicit: "*Appreciate
your heritage*.... A mark of maturity in any renewal movement is an ap-
preciation of its heritage. Kilian McDonnell warns against importing 'cultural baggage' from one religious tradition to another. By baggage he
meant styles of worship, speech mannerism, hymnody, pastoral and theological traditions."[3] To date most of the talk about healing has had to be a
borrowing. The movement is very busy finding more traces of impetus in
its own heritage. Meanwhile it argues for the legitimacy of importing practices from elsewhere, or recovering what it feels Lutheranism neglected—
so long as it is not opposed to the genius of a now thoughtless heritage.

Lutherans, of course, do not like to be discussed in terms of what they do
not believe, do not practice, do not have in their tradition. Precisely
because the charismatic approach to healing has not been constant or nor-
mative does not mean that it believes "less" but rather that it believes
"also" and "other." To illustrate this, I want to refer to a typical Lutheran
church body's inquiry into an aspect of healing. Deliberately, we shall
choose one from just before the outbreak of charismatic movements in
American Lutheranism. In 1960 and 1962 the large United Lutheran
Church in America in convention made a "long-term, intensive study" of
the entire field of anointing and healing. The United Lutheran Church
Board of Publication published it as *Anointing and Healing*.

Immediately, the drafters saw that they could not consider anointing in isolation from the whole concept of healing in the Lutheran church tradition. Health "theologically ... means salvation and healing means saving." But in their report, healing "becomes the restoration to normality of deranged physical and mental functions." Healing includes the contributions by members of the church "to scientific knowledge, psychological insight, medical skill, and human love. . . ." But what is *distinctive* about the church? The report acknowledges that dramatic healing *was* part of the New Testament church. It was allowed to fade in part because in the later church "Christian healing came to resemble healing miracles in the pagan world" and came to look superstitious, magical. "The impact of the Reformation meant a great reduction in the role of superstition and magic for the Christian community." Instead, Reformers restored the sacrament of the Lord's Supper as a forgiving, healing instrument.

Extravagant forms of healing went underground. But new times bring new urgencies. The authors argued that new understandings of science and nature were having a bearing on faith. "For the Christian believer what expectancy concerning healing is to be included in his faith in Christ?" Then follow important theological propositions. "Sickness as affliction is the result of the rebellion of the creature." This "does not imply a consistent causal connection between the afflictions of a given individual and his sin." Nor is bodily illness and death seen only as affliction. A number of christological comments follow. God healed in Jesus, and healing was a sign of the Kingdom, though it was not the only kind of sign.

The characteristic Lutheran response, the sort that draws the impatience and ire of charismatics, follows:

> Christ's injunctions to his disciples to perform such authoritative miracles were specific commissions for that time and circumstance, when the apostolic age marked a unique turning point in the history of redemption. Healing miracles are not part of any specified, Christ-commanded assignment for the on-going church.

When the church continued its healing work, this was part of its general ministry (*diakonia*) to the sick, "not ... a continuation of Christ's command to his disciples to perform miracles of healing." Yet healing, we read, may be part of the church's distinctive ministry in our day.

This Lutheran statement on healing reminds us that God "has many ways of healing only partially perceived by man." "Pain, sickness, therapy, and healing are important but secondary matters. They are penultimates." This claim recalls our opening comments about how for Lutherans these

are the second-best aspects of "well-being." One dare not confuse ulti-
mates with penultimates; one is cautioned, "When people attempt to use
faith in Christ to gain physical and mental health, they are making God's
grace the means toward some other end and are thus misusing the Gospel."
Then when "people talk of discovering spiritual laws that enable one to tap
Christ's supernatural powers for purposes of healing, they are misusing the
Law in an attempt to coerce God. These are attempts at magic."

Still, the denomination did not want to reject legitimate if extraordinary
approaches to healing and asked for what this book is asking: "The role of
history is carried by tradition (remembered history) and lives as a strong element in the church's present thought and practice." So tradition is a guiding
hand. The church must "start from the living tradition incorporated in present practice" and must approach healing critically. For the Lutheran tradition, many faith-healing claims "too easily engender a false expectancy concerning healing through faith in Christ." Yet Lutherans should not continue
to neglect penultimates such as bodily healing. Congregations should make
a much larger place for a "concern about the totality of each believer's life
that the burden of bodily sickness will be shared and will be met with concerned prayers." These provide an opening for spiritual healing when and
where God sees fit to heal through faith. Intercession for the sick has to be a
greater element in every congregation's life. The worshipers pray only with
"certainty in respect to God's will concerning a given sickness . . . that [God]
wills Christ's victory in this situation." Believers must be open to any signs of
that victory, also through bodily healing. And this intercession should go on
both in formal worship and in "small face-to-face 'enabling-groups' in
which the fellowship of the congregation becomes personal and envelops the
totality of the believer's life." If congregations are thus sensitive, "then we
can urge our members with real hope to turn in their need to their Lutheran
church rather than to 'faith healers.'"

EXPANSION OF TRADITIONS

The charismatic movement illustrates the theme that something fresh can
be brought into a tradition. The ULCA's *Anointing and Healing*, which
was pre- and partly anticharismatic, shows how the tradition exercises
control over excess, but its keepers are still prodded by challengers into extending the heritage and vivifying it. The accent on a form of "faith healing" that wants to be true to the Lutheran tradition will work chiefly in the
tradition of petitionary and intercessory prayer. Yet there may be some
borrowing here and there from those who advocate the use of oils, the laying on of hands, or participation in the charismatic movement.

Nevertheless, the report advises that "the use of oil in ministering to the sick would be unwise for our Lutheran congregations today." Here is an appeal to tradition: "Though such use of oil belongs to the living tradition of some other churches, it is not a part of the traditional practice of Lutherans." There is admitted biblical precedent in James 5:14, but "no direct application is possible because in Biblical times oil was thought to have medicinal value," and "there is danger that magical value would be attached to oil" or that it would seem like a new sacrament alongside the Lord's Supper. It is of interest that in 1982, in the major book of *Occasional Services* for Lutherans in America, an optional use of anointing oil was made available.

On the other hand—and who says Lutherans do not instinctively appeal to their tradition?—the ULCA report says that the "laying on of hands in ministering to the sick" is a sign of concern and blessing to be encouraged. Lutherans should discourage it only when "it readily suggests that through the hands are conveyed in a special way God's grace or God's healing power." Laying on of hands "belongs naturally in our tradition and society without adding a strange element and a new rite." It can be a "valued symbol—tangible and personalized for the sick—of a healing ministry."

The report comes to its climax and reposes in the tradition when it speaks of intercessory prayer. This has an integral place in worship, in Christian group life.

The characteristic and traditional Lutheran appeal to congregational life is clear and strong:

> ... Lutherans—and all who will heed this warning [should] be very careful about participating in efforts at spiritual healing that do not develop within the context of face-to-face Christian fellowship, a fellowship that is created first of all by the Gospel.

This is a concern about faith healers who confuse ultimate with penultimate matters and verge on quackery. "They fail to recognize as God's gift to man proven scientific methods and recognized therapeutic procedures." They "over-simplify faith and healing" and distort the image of serious people who stimulate faith and healing. "They endanger human lives." They "use the power of suggestion and mass hypnosis." These are serious charges, conventional in the literature before the mid-1960s in America.

After all the cautions in the report there comes the emphatic word: in Lutheran congregations "there should be much greater concern for sickness and health." But the authors do not spell out exactly *how* to express this.

Word about spiritual healing dare not become a new gospel. "The committee would not recommend the introduction of public services designated as healing services," since these could invite "misuse and misunderstanding." Yet in the ordinary services of worship, there should be some sort of healing emphasis.[4]

A demonstration of how intercession lives on in one part of the Lutheran tradition is in Peder Olsen's *Healing Through Prayer*. Olsen's book reflects the Norwegian tradition of a Pietism which is not charismatic but is also restless about the apathetic practice of prayer. After reviewing the biblical and ancient church lore, Olsen comes to the Reformation. Of course, the familiar Melanchthon incident appears, as does Luther's permission for the use of healing oils so long as they are not perceived sacramentally. As expected, Blumhardt also makes an appearance.

In order to amplify the tradition, Olsen refers to Wilhelm Löhe, a great nineteenth-century German Lutheran cleric who had a strong influence on the American church. At his Deaconess Home at Neuendettelsau, Löhe stressed healing through prayer:

> In order that the church might carry out its task in the world, the Lord has given it the gifts of the Spirit in the same way as Elijah gave Elisha his mantle. The special gifts of grace were given to the church on Pentecost. Have these gifts ceased to exist? No, it is only unbelief which holds this view. The Spirit is still present, and where the Spirit is there his gifts are also. It is possible to strive for these gifts, especially through prayer.

Notably in the mission field, where agents of Christian salvation and healing confronted "magical" and "pagan" views, Lutherans were called upon to stress healing with the laying on of hands and prayer. Olsen recalls a revival in Madagascar after 1894 under Rainisoalambo and his colleagues, "the Lord's disciples." An observer named Dr. Borchgrevink watched the revival as the sick were healed through prayer and the laying on of hands. He cited people cured of ovarian tumors, paralyzed arms, tubercular leprosy. "These people as well as the others who are healed have received faith to use the Word of God," said a medical doctor on the scene.

In his own Norway, Olsen typically bewailed the neglect of healing as a gift of grace "to the congregation," where it "has been little used and little considered by the men of the church, even though it *has always existed within the congregation*."(Emphasis mine.) He lauded a Pastor Vatne of Jaeren (d. 1941), who used anointing oil to good effect, and the more noted Professor Ole Hallesby, who also promoted such practices. Olsen, knowing of their contributions, expected an outpouring of response to the long-neglected gifts of healing. In America, "an anonymous survey among

Lutheran pastors indicated there was a considerable ministry of this kind going on without fanfare."[5]

Some of the most interesting extensions of the Lutheran tradition beyond Scandinavia, Germany, and America have been in the Third World. There Christians have had to stress healing as part of their medical mission and in the face of competition with natural healers or those once called "pagan." Typical of efforts to elaborate on the tradition in such settings was a Makumira Consultation held by the Evangelical Lutheran Church in Tanzania in 1967.

Although the original interest issued from the Lutheran church, many of the papers in the report were by Presbyterian John Wilkinson. Almost none of them drew explicitly on the Lutheran tradition, though they did implicitly reflect its concerns. Most delegates were from the Lutheran church, but most East African Christian agencies other than Roman Catholicism were represented. (Catholics had intended to participate.) The positive word about anointing oils came from Cuthbart K. Omari, of the Christian Council of Tanzania. He was not a Lutheran, but his cautionary words sounded Lutheran: "The act of anointing the sick with oil may be practiced, but we should remember that in the Bible it is not separated from prayer [and] we should be careful not to make this . . . into a magic act."

A reminder of how Lutheran and other Christian traditions collide with existing culture came in Lutheran Lloyd W. Swantz's essay on "local medicine," which reflected tribal lore and traditional medicine. He spoke appreciatively of the tradition in Africa. It uses the "family doctor," or *mganga*, who embodied very personal, not institutional, care. Traditional medicine recognizes the concept of the whole man, body and soul; did medicine in the West do as well? The *mganga* reunified the roles of doctor and pastor; should not the Western churches learn from this? There is group therapy; does the congregation, "the new 'tribe of God,'" do as well? Medical research shows much good in traditional medicine. Then comes the confrontation:

> Some Lutheran Synods/Dioceses in Tanzania even in official constitutions forbid Christians from using traditional medicines. These were written as if all local medicines had to be used with the blessings of a "witch-doctor" and mixed with superstition. Should not our constitutions and general thinking on this subject be reviewed, especially when we know in fact that 50–100% of the Christians and even the pastors are using local medicines? What burdens of guilt and conscience are perpetuated by such church laws or teaching? Is it not time to study anew the use of herbal medicine and also to clear the understanding and give warning on known bad medical and magical practices?[6]

Swantz might have been surprised to learn to what extent Lutheran synods and dioceses in America have seen the rise of "the Christians and even the pastors" exploring herbal medicines, health foods, natural dietary supplements, and the like. This brief visit to Tanzania illustrates once again the way a tradition is lived in flux, ever adapting, learning, while trying to be true to its genius. Christians in the West are learning this as they become aware of what goes on elsewhere.

·6·

Morality, Ethics, and Justice: Being Good and Being Well

At most points the human search for well-being involves morality and ethics. Whole encyclopedias have been written on the connection between mental or psychic health and the question of being good and doing good. Persons who depart from what their own value system has portrayed as "the good" may fail to be well because of the guilt produced by actions that do not match the values. The guilt may take form as neurotic anxiety. It may thus help generate illness instead of the very health the religion in question sets out to nurture.

CONNECTING MORALS WITH ETHICS: AN INVENTORY

The issue of personal morals is connected to that of ethical viewpoints and systems. What I consider to be good links somehow with what my elders, teachers, ministers, and other significant people have convinced me belongs to the tradition that is to guide me. This is the internal side of the way morality connects with well-being. But there is also an external connection. Whether or not I have a doctor who is a good person will have much to say about whether certain choices affecting me will go one way or another. It makes a difference whether or not I live in a society where people of good character and provident outlook are in control. This will help determine, for example, whether there will be hospitals to house me in illness and medical care systems that will prevent me from being financially devastated in the event of a catastrophe.

Persons who live in the world where moral questions affecting health and medicine are debated need no inventory of what the issues are. They could proceed at once to an examination of how people in a particular tradition live, are taught to live, or believe they should live. Most advice on well-being in America, however, still lies on the side of which toothpaste or tampon to use, which jogging method is best, or which form of health insurance is the most prudent purchase. So it is not feasible to assume that we are all talking about the same thing when we accent the role of religion, tradition, and church life on morality and ethics in medicine.

The *Encyclopedia of Bioethics* editors called upon John Ladd to define for them, as he shall for us, something of what is involved when the terms *ethics* and *morals* appear in connection with being well. Few agree on anything about the distinction between the two words except that *ethics* comes from the Greek and *moral* from the Latin. Ethics, in general can be

> taken to mean the philosophical inquiry into the principles of morality, of right and wrong conduct, of virtue and vice, and of good and evil as they relate to conduct. . . . "Ethics" is also sometimes used to refer to the beliefs or practices of a particular sect or group, as in Christian or Jewish ethics, or to describe the values or conduct of a particular individual, as in Hitler's ethics.

To the philosopher, ethics deals with "what . . . *ought* to be." To the historian of a tradition and thus to the author of this book, it also points to "what law is, or what custom is, or what institutions are, or what positive morality is." Thus we ask not only "What *should* Lutherans do?" but "What *do* Lutherans do?" in respect to being well or understanding health and medicine. There are, admits Ladd, "ethically significant connections between" *ought* and *is*.

Ethical questions and disputes rise for at least four reasons. First, there are "conflicts of interests." The Lutheran and the Jehovah's Witness have different interests. When the question of saving a child's life is concerned, if a blood transfusion is believed "medically" to be of help, the former supports and the latter forbids it. A patient has one set of interests that might collide with those of a nurse.

Second are "questions arising out of moral dilemmas." Shall we put more money into expensive care for people with catastrophic illness, for example those who profit from kidney dialysis, or more into improving the general health of thousands of the poor? Shall I as a physician cut off life-support systems and end some expense and misery but possibly violate the question of God's role or a patient's part in determining the hour of death? "Which of my prima facie duties ought I to perform when it is impossible to perform all of them?"

A third zone of dispute rises out of topics that relate to the present book: "ought-questions arising out of ethical disagreements." Says Ladd, "In a pluralistic society such as ours and in a world divided by different ideologies, religions, and cultures, it is inevitable that people should disagree over the rightness or wrongness of various kinds of conduct. An act that is regarded as right in one group is regarded as wrong in another group and as morally neutral in still another." The medical practitioner, Ladd writes, faces "moral problems" because he or she deals with people from competing traditions. Sometimes questions in this zone connect with moral dilemmas: "Does [a medical professional's] duty to respect the ethical beliefs of others that he knows to be wrong override his duty to save the patient's life?"

Fourth, there are "ought-questions turning on the distinction between duties and other oughts." It is not only "moral" questions that deal with morality. "It would be absurd to say that a doctor either has a duty to play golf on his day off or a duty not to do so, although it might be perfectly correct to say that he ought to play because he enjoys it." The problems can be more important than that one. For instance, "Why should a patient take pills prescribed by a doctor if he has no duty to try to get well?"[1]

DOING GOOD AND BEING WELL

Keepers of traditions know that morals and ethics in religion grow out of "rules and principles" those faiths teach. Thus Lutherans will say that their basic rules about being well and doing good grow out of divine law, especially as revealed in the Ten Commandments. They take absolutely seriously the absolute commands of Jesus. Their tradition has deduced certain rules that grow out of these.

Thus some say that abortion, the taking of fetal life, is explicitly forbidden by the commandment of God, "Thou shalt not kill." Rules have force. They also imply sanctions: the good Lutheran, some say, will not practice abortion and will try to effect legislation to prevent others from practicing it. Not to do so would lead one to be considered a bad member of such a Lutheran group. Other Lutherans would say that this is too concrete an application of a principle. Does "Thou shalt not kill" mean *never*? Then what about the Christian who cuts off a life-support system, fights in a war, or is a police officer?

The place of rules is a subject of heated debate within traditions, including the Christian and, within it, the Lutheran. Many would say that "rules" are secondary. They may describe the good life God intends. They may have a "political" use in the civil order. Yet, says this Lutheran tradition, though not all others do, keeping the rules will not "save" a person. It will not make him or her good *in the sight of God*. No human rule keeping, including in matters of taking or saving life, will be sufficient to merit the favor of God. God alone determines what is God pleasing. The Lutheran adds as a principle of her faith that "being well" before God and "doing good" are not so much acts of following rules but living by grace, realizing forgiveness, ac-

74334

cepting the gift of God's love in Christ. Moral and ethical life flow from the receipt of this gift. "The love of Christ" now controls believers. They will henceforth care about becoming channels of that love to others, for example to those in medical need. Or they will now care for their own bodies as "Temples of the Spirit," part of "the New Creation" in the resurrected Christ.

To a person in another tradition, this Lutheran "principle" as it relates to "rules" can be risky, even perverse. It may lead one to care for the life of a mother and thus to "kill" a fetus, even though there has been a prior rule against taking any life. Or the belief may mean interrupting a pattern of rules for the sake of healing. This was the case when Jesus "broke the Sabbath," a prescribed day of rest, in order to heal. Worst of all, it may breed "antinomianism" or lawlessness. In place of principle there could be the chaos of not caring about rules, since people may feel that, through forgiveness of sins *after*, ethical wrongdoing is so easily cleared from the divine slate. A "new being" comes forth daily, thanks to the works of God in Christ. So, reasons the believer, why should I take the rule seriously?

Few people live only by the "rules and principles" of their traditions. First, they cannot know what all of these are, or how to apply them. As Saint Paul reminded them, believers will not always have the will or the ability to carry out what they know these rules and principles impel them to do. Second, there may be a gap between what those rules and principles originally set forth and what they have become through the centuries. Thus, most Lutherans would be shocked to know all that is in early Lutheranism's value systems. Third, they have compromised many of these through the business of living in the passage of centuries.

Fourth, people pick up alien moral ideas from their environment. Some Lutheran oppposition to abortion may grow *not* out of Lutheran norms, but instead from contact with absolutists who claim a medical, scientific, philosophical, and theological knowledge about the status of fetal life that the tradition itself has not clearly spelled out. Other Lutherans draw their views on abortion less from their tradition of supporting life than from liberal views of freedom and the notion of a mother's self-determination or choice, as spelled out in twentieth-century situations. Yet it is valuable to check out moral and ethical life and thought in the light of the specific traditions, even though they may later be compromised or confused with other systems.

What we have done so far is suggest that "being well" does not come merely from aspirins, medical insurance, brushing one's teeth, or hoping that all will be well. It relates to choices one makes about what to do with one's own body and mind. And it is connected to what others think. "Doing good" and "being well" are fused along the way.

Second, we have shown that different systems of living or courses of life grow out of and produce competing ethical and moral outlooks and ways. Implied throughout is the worthiness of an examination of these traditions. Lutheranism stands within Protestantism, or "evangelical catholicism." Within Christianity, it has some distinctive flavors and stamps.

This is the point at which to confront a theme that haunts most pages of this book. Lutheranism is not "one thing," agreed upon by all Lutherans or their observers. It was one set of things in the sixteenth century, during the original ferment of Luther's reform. It was another in the seventeenth century, when people of a scholastic outlook schooled themselves in the art of "nailing things down," putting them in orthodox order. Lutheranism during the eighteenth century was again different, depending upon whether Pietism taught them to stress the heart and the will or Rationalism emphasized the mind. Lutheranism today keeps all these and many other elements in its cluttered mental attic.

Lutheran medical practices differ vastly depending upon whether they occur in a village hospital in Muslim Africa, a Lutheran hospital in America, or a secular setting in post-Christian Scandinavia. Technology, degrees of wealth, and cultural habits all help determine these differences.

Lutheranism also manifests differences as to what medical and health ethics and morals are in various cultures. There are gaps between what church leaders and theologians believe people *should* believe and what the people actually hold to as their faith system and ways of life. It is foolish to talk about "the Lutheran tradition" without becoming very aware of the many different ways this tradition influences the lives of Lutheran peoples.

Often, as author, I have pictured various kinds of Lutheran readers or non-Lutheran observers reading the pages of this book. One set of them may have grown up where legalism has turned Lutheranism into a very narrow, cramped, and crabby faith. The senior generation imparted rules and principles of a negative character. They succeeded in breeding mistrust of the body, of sexuality, of the physical world. To them these pages may now and then look like libertinism, liberation, or liberalism. The author portrays Lutheranism as a grace-filled, grace-full, dynamic tradition. That, some could say, does not square with the way Lutheranism looks and feels up close "where I came from."

Another set of readers, meanwhile, have grown up under pulpits where the Lutheran understanding of the gospel has played down rules and principles. What does matter is the immediacy of God's forgiving love in Christ. The zone and scope of freedom are very large. It is absurd to ask people to snuggle back "under the law" the way people in other traditions do. More often, we picture pages such as these catching the attention of people in very relaxed and slack "officially Lutheran" cultures such as those many Scandinavians find themselves occupying. They know Lutheranism is around them like a very loose envelope. At almost no point does it touch, bind, hold, or confine them. How could Lutheranism there be described as a tradition that has anything to say? Still others may live in a tiny Lutheran minority within a culture that belongs to others—to Muslims, Baptists, or, in many parts of America, pluralistically to "everybody and nobody." Such adherents are able to see few or no evidences of Lutheran power to set rules and principles.

A RANGE OF BELIEFS AND BEHAVIORS: THREE SAMPLES

A healthy dose of realism about a religious tradition enters, then, when we do some close-up looking at Lutheran cultures and subcultures. It is very hard to portray these accurately. We cannot follow unlabeled Lutherans into laboratories or medical schools, to say nothing of nurseries and bedrooms, to learn what their actual practices are. We can, it is true, measure something by seeing what they spend for hospitals, whether their congregations budget for human care, or what their birth and death rates are. That is some step up from mere hunches and guesswork or impressionism. Yet it is all still quite sketchy and subjective.

Scholars today find it possible to begin connecting belief and behavior, being well with doing good, theology or dogma and morals and ethics by linking such observation with opinion polling. The few surveys of this sort already taken offer promise and should inspire many more such surveys. Opinion polls, however, have their limits. The samples cannot be totally accurate. The questions may distort the answers, perhaps because they have to be overly precise. People often tell a poll taker something that they believe is expected from them rather than what they actually believe. The public has been suspicious of these surveys and sometimes has mistrusted their use, since some readers confuse statements about "is" with those urging an "ought." Yet, for all the hazards, we learn something instead of nothing and can use social scientific surveys to sketch something of what Lutheranism looks like ethically and morally today. Such a look will inspire modesty, especially among those who have thought that Lutheranism in its belief system generates a single response or way of life in all cultures. We shall pause to glance at Iceland and, in America, at Detroit and Minnesota.

Iceland

To make this issue of behavioral differences vivid, I want to consider in some detail, first, the extreme example of Iceland. That island nation may not be the center of many Lutherans' world, but it certainly belongs to the Lutheran world. Whoever thinks you can tell the whole story of a tradition only cognitively, by references to its dogma, its theology, and its thought patterns, will be confounded by a reality like that of Iceland. The people have been Christian since about the year 1000 and Lutheran for centuries, since the time the old nation changed along with its rulers. Both of these transitions were easy. Richard F. Tomasson, who made the most extensive opinion surveys and on whom we shall rely here, says that Icelanders have always been tolerant. "Few Icelanders have ever been intense pagans, intense Catholics, or intense Lutherans." Sugurdur A. Magnusson, a contemporary Icelandic writer, sees his people as "exceedingly tolerant in moral and religious affairs." Yet according to a survey taken in 1978, 97 percent of the people consider themselves "quite, somewhat, or slightly" religious.

Why is this so? Thórir Kr. Thórdarson, a theology professor at the University of Iceland, says that Lutheranism there was decisively shaped during the eighteenth century, the period of Rationalism. The "religious tradition [then] achieved a unity and strength never since equalled." The Icelanders were never subject to the Pietistic Awakenings that swept much of the Protestant domain in the eighteenth and nineteenth centuries. The citizens never acquired fervor; religion became a part of official life and it remains so.

In 1977, 97.2 percent of the population was Lutheran, with 93 percent of all the people belonging to the official church and only 4.2 percent to three Lutheran Free Churches. Only 1.6 percent were non-Lutheran affiliates in Catholicism, Adventism, Pentecostalism, and Bahaism. That left only 1.2 percent who made a point of no affiliation, according to the Statistical Bureau of Iceland. There are 110 clergymen, one for every 2,000 people. Church attendance probably varies from 1 to 2 percent of the population.

The Church of Iceland is liberal; Bishop Sigurbjörn Einarsson has said that "the liberalism associated with the turn of the century acquired greater and more lasting popularity . . . in Iceland than in Western European countries." What is more, the surveys show that Icelandic Lutheranism is also heavily tinged with occult beliefs; not all the old paganism disappeared. "Central to the belief system of modern Icelanders are all manner of psychic phenomena; prescience, foretelling the future; second sight; . . . the meaningfulness of dreams; . . . a belief that people can communicate with the dead or those absent. . . ." As for our medical topic, 41 percent had visited a faith healer, and 91 percent of these believed that they profited from the experience.

An area of health and well-being in which one can measure the moral and ethical norms of a faith has to do with sexuality, generation, familiarity, and the like. Tomasson's study shows a pattern of great tolerance or laxity in 97.7 percent Lutheran Iceland.

> Nowhere in the North has such long-term continuity been maintained in the area of marriage and sexual relations as in Iceland. Neither Latin Catholicism nor Lutheran, pietistic, or evangelical Protestantism ever overwhelmed the secular and egalitarian Germanic conceptions of the relations between the sexes that have remained tenaciously embedded in the folk culture of Iceland.

There is also a "remarkably tolerant view toward sexual relations." In Catholic days the clergy were not expected to practice celibacy. "No modern Western society, except [also Lutheran] Sweden, has approached Iceland's level of illegitimacy since the advent of modern vital statistics...."

Islands provide captive populations and neat boundaries. Social scientific surveyors therefore rub their hands in glee when they come across one. From within Iceland, Björn Björnsson's 1965 study drew most attention after he published it as *The Lutheran Doctrine of Marriage in Modern Icelandic Society*. He found "an awareness of somewhat unusual patterns of family organization" as he interviewed couples in Akranes, twenty miles from Reykjavik. Reluctant to ask intimate questions Björnsson found people volunteering intimate answers. These deviated from expected Lutheran moral and ethical norms, but the people "did not look upon their behavior as deviating in any sense...." Another researcher found that sexual questions produced less embarrassment than did economic ones.

Icelanders are great genealogists, and they publish elaborate tables. These trace back to certain key people. Thus, an example

> of the failure of orthodox Catholic views to subdue a certain early Norse "looseness" in things sexual as late as the sixteenth century is the case of Bishop Jón Arason (1484–1550) to whom virtually all Icelanders can validly claim direct descent. Jón was the last Catholic bishop of Iceland; he was beheaded by the Protestants for refusing to accept the "new faith." He had nine children with his concubine Helga Sigurdardottir.

In Lutheran times, "the clergy produced a not insignificant number of 'natural children,' with their paternity fully acknowledged and entered into the genealogical records." There are records of the illegitimacy of chil-

dren who later graduated under the theological faculty of the University of
Iceland between 1811 and 1931.

Hjalmar Lindroth wrote in 1937 that pre-Christian conceptions of life
lived on in Lutheran Iceland. "In pagan times such matters were hardly
moral questions at all, and still less religious in our sense, but social. . . .
Therefore a marked liberality and freedom from prejudice has always pre-
vailed in such things in Iceland." Similar conditions lived on well into the
nineteenth century in Norway and Sweden. Illegitimacy rates went down
in those Scandinavian areas most touched by Pietism, evangelical awakenings, and revivals, says Tomasson.

Women have always had a higher status in liberal Lutheran Iceland
than in more orthodox and Pietist nations, and divorce was not stigmatized.
The Icelanders are also "the most unmarried of all the Scandinavians," but
"a sizable proportion of Icelanders continue to cohabit in relationships of
varying duration and stability, as they have for centuries."

Another one of the issues of health and medicine that scholars can
measure better than others and one that many religionists have connected
with morals and ethics is the use of alcohol. Iceland has severe problems
with alcohol, expensive though it is. The occasions for drinking are fewer
than in some other nations, but people know few restraints. Icelanders
drink more at more risk to life and limb than do citizens of many other nations. Traffic offenses involving alcohol are much more frequent than in
most Nordic countries. "Sporadic excess is an apt description of the pre-
dominant drinking patterns of Icelanders." Of course, there has also been
a strong temperance movement and for a time "total prohibition," which
ended when the Spanish refused to buy Icelandic fish if the Icelanders did
not buy Spanish wine.

As for the official guardians of ethics and morals, Tomasson writes:

> There is one section of the population that has been particularly prone to
> drunkenness: the clergy. During the years 1741–1745, Ludvig Harboe,
> the clergyman sent by the Danish king to investigate the ability of Icelan-
> dic youth to read and their knowledge of Christian teachings, found a
> number of the priests, who should have been teaching the young, to be
> drunkards.

Later observers for a long period regularly observed the same. There
may now be some new health and moral consciousness; "in the twentieth
century . . . members of the clergy have not been particularly noted for
their tippling, just as they are no longer noted for their fathering of illegiti-
mate children."

Do deviations from sexual and familial moral norms or overindulgence in alcohol disturb the people of Iceland? If they are Lutherans, they are supposed to be possessed with a drive for forgiveness, based on a repentance that is located next to guilt. If Tomasson and the people he cites are accurate, Iceland remains at the left end of the Lutheran spectrum and believers show only a fuzzy sense of the tradition in their actions:

> . . . The Icelanders are an extremely tolerant people. They manifest a tolerance in moral, religious, and intellectual matters that is pervasive and goes deep. . . . Perhaps this tolerance is related to the strong communal nature of the Icelanders and their strong primordial sentiments, which are similar to the feelings people have toward kin.

They also fear making enemies; "the person one offends today may be one's in-law or workmate tomorrow." Theologically,

> another factor is that Iceland is more a "shame culture" than a "guilt culture." "Guilt cultures" prevail in Western societies in which Christianity is more deeply rooted than in Iceland. Icelanders do not want to confess their sins—they just do not want anybody to know about them. They do not have guilt feelings to project into others.[2]

Iceland is a special case, of course. It may strike Lutherans in pluralist America as a mere curiosity. The United States, including its Lutherans, has been heavily influenced by Puritanism, Pietism, evangelical revivals, awakenings, and moralistic movements. The Lutheran church is a minority that has little chance to shape the whole culture, though its strong congregations can help mold both subcultures and individuals. In America the Lutherans have shown far more interest in following historic Lutheran norms. At the same time, great gaps exist between what the clergy teach and what people think Lutheran Christianity is about and expects of them. We shall visit two more samples to illustrate the issue of "living tradition" as opposed to mere book knowledge of dogma past in respect to ethics and morals.

Detroit

There are many thousands of Lutherans in metropolitan Detroit. They are almost lost in the pluralism of the city and suburbs and have not shaped the larger environment. In the late 1960s an ambitious survey there measured Lutheran attitudes toward belief and morals. The result was a set of findings that points to much more congruence between historic Lutheran traditions and practices than in, say, Iceland. At the same time it demonstrates gaps between belief and practice, between clergy and laity, when it comes to many of our "well-being" topics.

The author, Lawrence K. Kersten, consulted theologians and took pains to spell out a Lutheran ethic that differed from both Catholicism and Calvinism. He stressed the Lutheran accent on the Fall, on human powerlessness and the bondage of the will, and the free gift of grace in Christ.

> The present study reveals little uniformity in beliefs about the original nature of man among the clergy and laity of the four branches of Lutheranism. In fact, in regard to most all beliefs, a single, unified Lutheran Weltanschauung does not exist in the United States.

He did find more correlation between conservative theology and conservative politics, or between liberal Lutheran theology and liberal politics, than within Lutheranism across the spectrum of theology or politics.

On the crucial and central Lutheran theme, the clergy have either not been articulate or they have not been heard.

> Although Lutheranism is usually considered to be a religion stressing the grace of God rather than the Law of God . . . the majority of Lutheran laymen today, in contrast to their views of being saved by God's grace through faith and trust, also say that they are saved by keeping the Ten Commandments and living a good moral life. Luther's strong emphasis on the Law of God thus exists today despite the contradictory evidence of theology. A stress on moral conduct, based on Old Testament Law, is almost as much a part of the thinking of the individual Lutheran layman as is the concept of free grace.

We have argued that Lutherans see themselves more as a caring community than an agency of social change, more ready to support charities than to work for social reform and a welfare society. The Kersten study bears this out emphatically and here finds more connection between Lutheran teaching and practice.

> In keeping with Luther's definition of the role and function of the church as "preaching the gospel," most Lutherans surveyed oppose efforts for social reform by the church. Little in Lutheran theology directs the church to attempt to build the kingdom of God in this world. . . . In its emphasis on philanthropy and charity rather than social reform, Lutheranism tends to "alleviate but not recreate." Such thinking is harmonious with the traditional Lutheran doctrine of the two kingdoms.

The Detroit Lutherans were ready to feel that "works should follow from grace" in *personal* moral conduct. They also thought, however, that "no collective efforts toward social reform are considered desirable or necessary." The more liberal clergy and the black Lutherans deviated most from this. They favored Lutheran social action. Many others felt that Lutherans should make little effort at all to change the social order. Presumably, this would mean that if the economic system prices medical care out of the reach of the poor, or society does no regulating of nursing homes, Lutherans would not work as Lutherans to change the situation. They may try to help the poor or visit the aged. Perhaps, as individuals apart from the church, they might agitate or legislate, shall we say, "secularly." A Lutheran teaching that people should be content within their lot and calling seems to outweigh impulses to organize for change.

Another dimension of the Lutheran ethic bearing on health that Kersten measured was its support of secular institutions, such as government and social organizations. "Whatever the existing situation of the social order, man can be assured that it has its good side, inasmuch as it is a product of God's will." So Lutherans tend to be submissive to these institutions. The great if biased social philosopher Ernst Troeltsch saw much in understanding "the beginning of social impotence of Lutheranism, in so far as it had not adopted Calvinistic and modern ideas." Thus in Detroit the surveyed Lutherans overwhelmingly disapproved of civil disobedience. That subject may be remote from medical concerns, yet on the horizon is the possibility of civil disobedience by conservative Christians, who have Lutheran allies, on the subject of laws dealing with abortion and other aspects of moral life in America.

One evidence of change in response to the Lutheran tradition, according to Kersten, had to do with well-being within the family. Yet Lutherans characteristically show caution in embracing the news of the changing:

> Despite the fact that the Lutheran ethic provides a patriarchal orientation toward family life, Lutherans today feel that women should have as much to say as men in both the family and the church. However, with the exception of the theologically liberal clergymen, other aspects of traditional Lutheran theology, such as an emphasis on obedience in childrearing and opposition to premarital and extra-marital sexual relations, still receive strong support. On the other hand, only the theologically conservative clergymen follow Luther's negative views regarding birth control and divorce.

By the late 1960s, there was even much wavering among them on birth control.

Medical searches for well-being today include the almost unquestioned acceptance of evolutionary theory in biology as a basis for research. "The data show that Lutherans today, except for theologically liberal clergymen, hold to non-scientific views regarding the origins of man and also see serious conflicts between science and religion."

Kersten perhaps too readily follows Troeltsch and Max Weber in their understanding that "the Lutheran ethic offers no real unified moral or ethical system," but he is probably correct in one dimension:

> The primary moral obligation is absolute self-surrender in faith and trust to God. Luther disliked emphasizing behavior or morality because it seemed to border on good works. As far as he was concerned, attempts to externalize religion into laws, rules, and regulations only degrade it. This study supports the conclusion that the Lutheran ethical system is one of individual morality and piety. No group or communal concern is evident, the result being a strong emphasis on religious individualism. . . . The consequences of these ethical ideas are reflected in the social impotence of Lutheranism in the entire secular realm. . . . Pietistic indifference, which the Lutheran conception of the two kingdoms emphasizes, expresses itself in the lack of basic ethical commands in the world.

Several of Kersten's specific findings flesh out his summaries. His fifth chapter is "Religion and Morality," our subject. Many of its topics have a bearing on the themes of being well. Kersten worked out a scale by comparing the four major Detroit area synods—LCA (Lutheran Church in America), ALC (American Lutheran Church), MS (Missouri Synod), and WS (Wisconsin Synod)—thus running from what many regard as being most liberal to most conservative. To take a comparatively trivial question, social dancing, Kersten can point to great changes. Not many years ago moderate-through-conservative Lutheranism saw dancing to be immoral and unhealthy. There were threats to morality in the surroundings, debauchery, costume, hours, and ways of life accompanying social dancing. The conservative clergy have by now lost their battle to oppose dancing. Today few laymen oppose it. Ninety-five percent of the LCA and ALC, 90 percent of the WS, and 89 percent of the MS laymen say it is not wrong. Only 56 percent of the MS clergy and 7 percent of the WS clergy give a response to match that of their people!

Smoking has only recently become an issue of health and morals. Opposition to it has had to make its way against a long Lutheran tradition of neutrality on smoking. Here we notice a curious twist, perhaps because opposition to smoking comes in part from secular and liberal (environmental, political) forces. Although the link between smoking and ill health is so widely accepted as to be unchallenged outside the tobacco industry, as recently as the late sixties "approximately 50 percent of the LCA, ALC, and MS clergy and 60 percent of the WS clergy do not see smoking as wrong." Is it always wrong? Only 19 percent of the LCA, 7 percent of the ALC, 6 percent of the MS, and 0 percent of the Wisconsin Synod thought so. "Thus the clergymen from the theologically most liberal Lutheran body are more likely to see smoking as a moral issue than the clergymen from the theologically most conservative body." More lay people than clergy believed smoking was always wrong. "Nearly half the clergymen say that they smoke, a factor which may explain their attitudes." Much theology is packed into that terse comment!

While the divorce rate was going up and Christian resistance to some of the implications of divorce was going down, the Detroit Lutherans moved very cautiously in changing their views. In all four synods, clergy were more ready than laity to agree that "although never a totally satisfactory answer to family problems, divorce is often the best solution." Clergy are consistently more liberal than laymen about attitudes toward performing the marriage of a divorced person. Here our assumptions about the pastoral "softening" of a harsh Lutheran ethic may be confirmed.

In specific matters of sexual well-being and understanding, "the Lutheran ethic strongly condemns homosexuality." The survey did occur before the recent increase in public awareness of and debates about homosexuality, so the attitudes may well have changed by now. In the late 1960s Kersten posed the statement, "Homosexuals are to be condemned and should be put in prison." How did the laity answer? Twenty-two percent in the ALC, 32 percent in the LCA, 34 percent in the MS, and 38 percent in the WS agreed. As for clergy, 8 percent in the LCA, 11 percent of the ALC, 22 percent of the MS, and 75 percent of the WS agreed.

On the subject of premarital and extramarital sex, Kersten accurately summarizes the traditional view: "The Lutheran ethic prescribes that premarital and extramarital sexual relations are explicitly and unquestionably wrong." Lutherans continue to hold generally conservative views on such subjects. Only a small percentage of those sampled favored sexual relations even with the person one intends to marry. How does all this relate to well-being? "Although the clergy percentages are somewhat larger, in every lay and clergy group the majority see serious emotional problems arising from premarital sex." Could a particular situation ever justify extramarital relations? "In the four clergy groups 44 percent of the LCA, 30 percent of the ALC, 17 percent of the MS, and 6 percent of the WS clergy agree that it might."

One of the more openly debated issues of well-being and marital health has to do with the expression of sex within marriage. In recent years conservative church groups, perhaps to compensate for the lures of extramarital sex in the culture or to give expression to more ample biblical views, have accented the theme of variety and abandon in marital sexual expressions. In 1967 Kersten asked for people to agree or disagree with the statement: "Because of the religious nature of marriage, sexual relations between husband and wife should be carried out with restraint." The findings? Thirty-two percent of the ALC and 42 percent of the MS agree that they should. Thus, over one-third of the laity think that restraint in sexual intercourse is appropriate even after marriage. The student generation deviated widely from this and showed their support for absence of restraint.

Kersten worries about issues of health and well-being on this subject.

> The previous data suggest that the attitudes of many Lutherans toward sex may be so rigid as to hinder normal sexual relationships in married life.... Many Lutherans may harbor considerable guilt about sexual matters. All societies, of course, must have rules governing sexual behavior. But if the rules are too harsh or produce extensive guilt, then perhaps a reevaluation is necessary.

Is change in a tradition then permitted or advisable? When asked whether "traditional religious standards" in sex relations "are no longer adequate, laymen decisively disagree." The clergy show vast differences in opinion, with 27 percent in the LCA and 94 percent in the small WS wanting no change. "A liberal theological position apparently engenders acceptance of a more liberal sexual code." As for the Lutheran clergy, when asked to react to the phrase "the unchanging Law of God is an absolute standard by which to measure man's conduct," a spectrum of Lutheran ethics appeared. Forty-five percent of the LCA, 69 percent of the ALC, 87 percent of the MS, and 100 percent of the WS agree.

Should "good sex education in high school . . . include knowledge on methods of birth control"? Among the clergy, only 15 percent of the LCA and ALC disagreed, but 88 percent of the WS did. Abortion, already then debated but not nearly so brutally as it has been since the Supreme Court *Roe* v. *Wade* decision, may have caught the Lutheran laity off guard. "A woman should have the right to get an abortion if she does not want to bring a child into the world." There were great differences of response. Disagreements came from 67 percent of the LCA, 71 percent of the ALC, 75 percent in the MS, and 80 percent of the WS. As for clergy, 57 percent of the LCA, 82 percent of the ALC, 92 percent of the MS, and 100 percent of the WS ministers disagreed.

Fortunately for our purposes, the Detroit survey also asked an institutional question. The Lutherans there were very individualistic about mor-

ality, yet they were also loyal members of congregations. These congregations can be instruments of care. Do you disagree with this statement? "All Lutheran congregations should contribute to the support of certain forms of ministry in the city such as to skid row people, hospitals, the aged or youth?" As for the laity, only 7 percent of the LCA, 4 percent of the ALC, 12 percent of the MS, and 29 percent of the WS disagreed. Clearly, they thought there should be such responsibility. Curiously, the clergy were more cautious in the Wisconsin Synod, where 50 percent disagreed, but elsewhere laity and clergy overwhelmingly supported this institutional role for congregations.

What about issues of priorities? Here was another question: "The primary responsibility of the local congregation is to serve the needs of its membership before serving the needs of those outside the church." Do you agree? Yes came from 67 percent of the LCA, 67 percent of the ALC, 76 percent of the MS, and 78 percent of the WS laity. There was an impressive difference here in lay and clergy figures. Clergy agreement was only 27 percent in the LCA, 35 percent in ALC, 45 percent in MS, and 50 percent in WS. "In summary, Lutheran laymen more than the clergy see the local congregation as serving its own members before providing for the needs of those outside the church." The more people are involved in "the Lutheran sub-community," the less human need beyond their own do they see.

In recent years the more liberal American Lutheran church bodies have issued denominational statements on social issues, including those having to do with abortion, birth control, death and dying, and other aspects of care. The Lutheran ethic traditionally did not prepare members for such action. How does it stand today? Should there be such statements? As for laity, yes say 45 percent of the LCA, 43 percent of ALC, 40 percent of the MS, and 30 percent of the WS. The clergy generally rank them much higher: 95 percent and 87 percent in LCA and ALC, 62 percent in MS support them, but only 13 percent in the WS do. As for social action in general, the more liberal clergy outrank all others in believing that the Lutheran ethic impels Christians into that sphere.[3]

Minnesota

Symbolically, but not geographically, somewhere beyond Iceland and Detroit lies Minnesota, the state with more Lutherans than any other in the United States. Fortunately for surveyors, there is considerable distribution among Lutheran synods in that state, with the Lutheran Church in American predominating and the moderate American Lutheran Church and the more conservative Missouri Synod generously flanking it. In the early 1980s the Institute for Cultural and Ecumenical Research at College-

ville, Minnesota, undertook a study to be published as *Faith and Ferment*.
Billed as the most extensive regional opinion survey of faiths to date, this
study does show how Minnesotans feel about matters of faith and morals.
Many of them have a bearing on health, medicine, and understandings of
being well.

The study found that "artificial birth control and family planning are an
accepted part of the Lutheran moral grid (84 percent)." Nor do many (22
percent) find abortion always wrong or sinful. But 64 percent reject premarital sex and 86 percent denounce extramarital sex. In their moral patterns homosexuality is not easily accepted; 64 percent find it "immoral"
and 35 percent say that it is "regrettable" or at best "permissible." Slightly
over half of the Lutherans think that sex education in schools should be
mandated.

Where do these Minnesota Lutherans get their ideas of moral norms?
Over 90 percent see the Bible as the authoritative word of God. Some 36
percent think that all the teachings of the church are essential to faith, but
the other 64 percent say that whether they hold to specific teachings of the
church or not, they have a deep faith. About half (53 percent) call the Lutheran "the true church" of Christ. Although 78 percent believe that people are sinful and 72 percent think of themselves as sinful, they are not radical Lutherans. Only 43 percent think that "an innate tendency to sin, and
not simply circumstances, is responsible for evil."

On social issues, as was the case in Detroit, many—in fact most—did not
think the church should concern itself *as* church to exert leadership in social justice issues. Only 45 percent were ready for that. Fewer (36 percent)
believe that true Christianity requires that the poor and oppressed be liberated or that Christianity requires a change in American society itself (29
percent). We can see again from this that if better health care or delivery
demands some structural change in America, the Lutherans give few signs
of being ready to work for it. They were not opposed to technology; at least
49 percent thought that at the present time a Christian way of life implies
the discriminating use of technology to make life better.[4]

A SUMMARY VIEW

If we keep the Icelandic end of the spectrum out of view—it served chiefly
to show how "folk" religion lives on in spite of centuries of Christianization, or to show that cultural change can overwhelm faith distinctives—a
profile begins to emerge from these and other studies. Among the fairly
consistent themes in the Lutheran tradition, the following are observable
in American debate and life.

1. The *universal priesthood* of believers has gradually been translated into an individualized, personal, and *private ethic*. Lutherans tend to see themselves "on their own," as it were, responsible for their conduct but not necessarily able to do much about the society or culture in general.

2. Alongside the universal priesthood and individualism, the *congregation* matters most as the communal form of faith. From it people get their norms, or think they do; through it they express much of their concern for well-being.

3. The Lutheran tradition has been maladept at fashioning generations of people who can see a reason or a means for *changing the social order* or removing evils and injustices in it as steps toward improving human well-being. They have not found a mechanism—denominational statements, social action, or others—that might fairly convey ways for the church to act in the world.

4. Lutherans compensate for their meager understanding or lack of action in the field of social justice by wanting to see themselves and be seen as *caring*, effecting works of charity, as individuals and in congregations.

5. They like to think of themselves as getting their norms from the Bible and Lutheran teachings, though their *actual beliefs* might deviate considerably from what theologians contend these documents mandate.

6. In general Lutherans tend to be conservative, advocating *"go-slow"* policies for changing institutions or adapting to new values. If something from the past is good and workable, it is held to. The passion for novelty seen in the more liberal church is less vivid and visible in this tradition.

7. In matters of *sexual morality*, extra- and premarital sexual intercourse tend to be prohibited. There has been some moderation of old stands against homosexuality and divorce. On some issues, however, there has been drastic change: "artificial birth control" and dancing, both of which not long ago were abhorred by most Lutherans, now gain wide justification.

8. In controversial matters, Lutherans expect and exhibit a *pastoral* stance. That is, they seek to keep a rule or principle, but they do not want it applied legalistically, heartlessly, or impersonally. Care for the well-being of the person may sometimes force relaxation of a rule.

9. There are great gaps between what the *clergy* think they are teaching and what they hold, and what the *laity* think they are being taught and what they hold. Lutheran clergy have not been very successful at getting Lutheran distinctives, including the central teaching about grace, across to their members.

10. There are *differences between various strands* of Lutheranism. Conservative Missouri and Wisconsin, the two synods that are not going

into the creation of a united new Lutheran church, are more tenacious about resisting cultural and theological change. Clergy, and to a lesser extent laity, in the other two Lutheran bodies are more ready for change, more open to receiving secular or ecumenical impulses.

11. There is some concern for seeing *the body* and care for it as theological and religious necessities. Although Lutherans divide life between understandings of God's "proper" work, to save one, and God's extended work, to provide order, care of the body is growing into a theological issue.

12. Evidently, a Lutheran understanding of *vocation* or the calling is widespread and motivates egalitarian views of spiritual potential in various fields of service, in medical professions as well as in Christian ministry.

13. The social scientists tend to draw on Ernst Troeltsch and Max Weber for their definitions of what classic Lutheran ethics has been. Therefore, they *overestimate* the theological theme of Lutheran "passivity" and "impotence" in the area of social change. They thus overlook a half century of research into the meanings of Luther and Lutheranism.

14. The surveys suggest that it will be fruitful for congregations and individuals to engage in selective retrieval of elements from their *tradition*. At the very least, members should have to confront their church's ethical and moral teaching, even if in the end they depart from some of its approach. The Lutheran tradition, that is, needs correction by examination of its own roots, original statements, and weathered intentions.

15. Despite these consistencies, Lutheranism is a *broad and diverse* tradition with many competing and sometimes mutually exclusive accents in the fields of morals and ethics.

A SAMPLE OF INQUIRY ON DEATH

American Lutheran denominations have entered the debate on moral and ethical questions. They want to bring both belief and behavior under scrutiny. Church bodies publish works on Lutheran views of ethics. They now charter commissions to study significant moral issues in the field of well-being. Sometimes the issues move beyond task forces and conferences. They become voted-upon statements of what a Lutheran denomination in general has to say about an issue. Abortion, homosexuality, death and dying—all these have provoked Lutheran moral and ethical comment. Some of the pronouncements are self-consciously Lutheran in that they seek sources and resources in the roots of the tradition. Others merely express the voices of Lutherans as they draw upon the Bible, the history of Christian ethics, and ecumenical and secular thought in general.

This is not the place to anthologize, collate, analyze, or criticize these documents. An example will illustrate the character of moral and ethical reasoning that goes with such inquiries. Since the visits to Iceland, Detroit, and Minneapolis—the *is* paragraphs—have dealt with sexual ethics, this sample of *ought* language will relate to another motif, the cessation of being. The Lutheran Church in America in convention in 1982 culminated a rather intense study of death and dying by approving a statement on the theme.

The statement begins with an observation on technology in the contemporary world. It points to achievements of medicine in the fields of organ transplants, dialysis machines, vaccines, and other means of prolonging life. "The irony of modern medicine is that with the new technologies that vastly expand the range of what it is possible to do has also come the anguish of deciding when it is appropriate to use these capabilities." Nowhere, the document argues, are these more pressing than in respect to death and dying. These situations present "new and difficult moral decisions that call for prayerful reflection and the support of a caring community."

Showing that they belong in the Lutheran tradition, these representatives of a church body do not expand on the technical analysis. Nor do they draw on philosophy, discuss rules and principles, point to utilitarianism or the categorical imperative. Instead, they move at once to theology. That theology points them to "biblical origins and ... subsequent development." Each theme—death as natural, death as tragic, death as friend, death as enemy—calls forth specific biblical citations. The principle for selecting these citations, even when not so stated, tends to be Lutheran. The informed Lutheran will recognize the author's preference for Saint Paul's language concerning baptism in Romans 6 and an interpretation Lutherans associate with baptism.

On this biblical-theological basis members are asked not to be content with mere "situation ethics," "new morality," or simple spontaneity. Instead, they are to reflect carefully and prayerfully in the immediate situation. Then "Scripture, *tradition*, and the shared reflection of Christian people will provide important resources." [Emphasis mine.] The statement proposes a set of "interpretive principles" that help determine believers' responses. Some of these will be familiar to those in the Lutheran tradition even if not everyone in Iceland or Detroit has picked them up. Thus the principle that "both living and dying should occur within the context of a caring community" takes precedence over privatistic views. Yet the person in every case matters greatly: "A Christian perspective mandates respect for each person" and his or her preferences. There must be concern for all who make decisions: the patient, physician, close family, pastor, and other members of the health care team. Hospital ethics committees are to be called on with more eagerness and hope than courts of law should be.

On these stated grounds, this Lutheran reflection on death and dying then proposes some circumstances in which treatment might be withheld or withdrawn. These include the case of "the irreversibly dying patient," "burdensome treatments," and "chronically ill individuals." Each presents very different ethical problems. Care could not be withdrawn from the chronically ill except in some hard-to-foresee, extreme situations. The church body also went on record against "active euthanasia." Where intended end of life ensues in a form that seems close to suicide, "it is also crucial that the Christian community not forget its responsibilities to minister to family members and other survivors."

Meanwhile, there must always be service to those who survive the critically ill, dying, or dead person. To make their point in a distinctive way, the statement draws on a Lutheran understanding of "the sacramental ministry of the church." This ministry includes "remembrance of baptism." Such a theme is dearer to Lutherans than to many other Christians in the contexts of therapy. The chapters of the statement also urge that recognition must be given to the humanity of health care professionals, who are frequently asked to bear tremendous burdens. They may need grief-therapy sessions and other signs of care.

The statement almost reflexively ends with a section on forgiveness and thanksgiving. A general statement on death and dying would need no such conclusion. Other Christian traditions might pick up some other theme. This one is Lutheran.

> There is much that we do not know.... In responding to the dilemmas that are thrust upon us in death-and-dying situations, we sometimes make the wrong decision, or at least are uncertain as to whether we have made the right one. And we are often woefully inadequate in extending compassion and understanding to our fellow human beings. Even in the best of circumstances, our sins and shortcomings are manifold.
>
> But this we know: God is merciful and forgiving. Thus, by grace, we can both experience forgiveness and forgive others, as God forgives us.

An implementing resolution added to the document helps guide individuals, congregations, the national church, hospitals, nursing homes, other health care institutions. At no point do the words *Luther* or *Lutheran* appear. Theoretically, another Christian body could have said much the same, though the sacramental views would not match those in Baptist, Free Church, or many Calvinist forms of Protestantism that make up the

American majority. The accent on all the pages falls not on absolute rules but on biblical witness and on sober reflection in trying circumstances. The statement is not highly controversial; it is an attempt to absorb extremes. Such terms as "active euthanasia" or "never intervene" would have been controversial alternatives. The chapters seek to help make it possible for Lutherans to think and act without total ignorance, darkness, fear, or guilt.[5] Here is another example of the tradition in action.

THE CASE OF THEOLOGY AND ETHICS

Documents from a Lutheran Church in America's inquiry on "Biomedical Ethics: Theological Perspectives" early in the 1980s carries conscious reference to the Lutheran tradition. The timetable for study of this document matched that proposed for death and dying.

> The Lutheran Church in America is a Christian community in which traditions and hopes, faith and commitments are nurtured and sustained. Its theology and morality have taken shape in historical circumstances. . . . Its members are affected by the current biological and medical events. . . . They are also influenced by its theology and moral teachings.
>
> The Lutheran tradition has accented some themes in our common human and Christian heritage that are of particular relevance as we reflect on the challenges. . . .

In other words, the church should have no interest in Lutheran sectarian uniquenesses, but on distinctive emphases within the larger Christian heritage. The statement specifies many of these while documenting particulars thence from the Lutheran tradition.

> The Lutheran understanding of divine law affirms that there are limiting conditions which humans must respect. They are formulated as a result of reflection, experience and, in science, by inquiry and experimentation. . . . Laws have an historical character. At certain moments in time these limits are boundaries that must be respected. . . . The boundaries change. . . . Once we had to accept our genetic fate, now we can alter it. . . . Our alterations are not made without the risk and pain of failure, but they are made.

A whole section on "God Redeems," without mentioning it, affirms the Lutheran tradition's way of looking at the divine-human grace relation. After a creedal summary, the statement moves to the "social setting for stewardship." It begins, "The Lutheran tradition affirms a strong respect for the social settings within which faithful stewardship is exercised." And the Lutheran understanding of vocation is clear:

> ... Christian stewardship is not confined to religious activities ("church work") but is exercised in secular stations of service within social structures such as (or including) the scientific and medical establishments. In these structures the incentives of mutual trade-offs (exchanges) of services and supplies and the disciplines of rules and laws prompt and prod humans to work for the common good.

Those dependent upon scholars Ernst Troeltsch and Max Weber but who are uninformed by the later recovery of the more ample Lutheran tradition, would say that the accents on "social action" belong to liberal clergy and do not represent the outlook of the bulk of the laity. Perhaps. Here may be a case of the authors reaching deeper into the tradition in their desire to instruct the church at large.

> Although the emphasis is on the beneficial functions of these structures, it is also recognized that such institutions can become powerful and consolidated forces of evil which obstruct positive achievements and destroy mutual human exchanges.

> Service in these systems must be given with a sense of critical judgment. The duty of social criticism is implicit in the Lordship of Christ and the way of the cross. The time comes when it is necessary to engage in controversy and struggle for positive gains on the edges of human development. Lutheran social ethics allows for coercive action but the emphasis is on responsibility for using methods of argumentation and persuasion whenever possible.

The statement wants Lutherans to stop standing on the sidelines with their theology. They should cooperate wherever "common criteria of judgment based on empirical evidence and rational thought can be discerned." There is room here for "civil righteousness." This is a form of serving God that does not help assure salvation. Instead, it improves human life and public order. Of course, there is also to be repentance "by which we correct our aim and course in our vocation as God's deputies."

In such paragraphs a billboard marked "Lutheran" could not better signal the presence of the tradition. To place such a billboard, however, would violate the statement's antisectarian impulse. There are some less explicit Lutheran accents in subsequent paragraphs on "wholeness," "autonomy," "nonmaleficence," "beneficence," "justice," and "veracity."[6]

Whether or not a reflective church in Iceland would come up with accents such as these, we do not know. They very consciously reflect a generation of fusion between experts in biomedical ethics and Lutheran theological understandings. One could illustrate further with similar statements from the other major Lutheran bodies. They would include emphatic statements on abortion and human sexuality by conventions or panels of the Lutheran Church–Missouri Synod. Such documents may not satisfy members of other Lutheran bodies. They cannot represent everyone within each speaking church body. But they do result from a process designed to make the tradition active. Statements by Unitarians, fundamentalists, agnostics, idealists, and presumably even of Calvinists and Roman Catholics—the nearest partners to Lutherans in medical ethics—would presumably pick up different accents.

A LUTHERAN STUDY OF CARE AND HEALING

All the fine talk about theological resources in morals and ethics is meaningless unless it is enacted. The Lutheran Church in America, further pursuing the resources of the Lutheran tradition, charged one of its divisions to find ways of nudging Lutherans into action. It chose Ralph Peterson to draft such a nudge, which he completed in January 1982. The result was *A Study of the Healing Church and Its Ministry: The Health Care Apostolate*.

Peterson took his assignment seriously and, some would say, took Lutheranism a bit over-seriously. He reminded readers that religious institutions formed by far the largest network of voluntary associations in American society. Yet this fact is often overlooked. There has to be recovery of their traditions. Then the Peterson trumpet sounded:

> The Lutheran Churches, more than any other denomination, have provided important national leadership in the health field. Fritz Norstad and Granger Westberg urged the church to "get back into health care" decades ago. It is only recently that many of us have really understood the scope of their vision.

The author cited agencies such as the Wheat Ridge Foundation and the Institute of Human Ecology of Lutheran General Hospital in Illinois as examples. He spoke of "the potential contribution from Lutheran initiative for a renewed understanding of a health ministry in our country. . . . Once again we must connect with the tradition."

This LCA statement inventoried some Lutheran moral and ethical teachings. It presented a fifteen-point charge to the Lutheran church and suggested nine projects. Most of them focused on beginning in "a state or region with a strong tradition of Lutheran mission in social ministry," "a strong Lutheran medical center," such as a theological school, institutes, and the like. Tradition, we are reminded, is not just talk but inspiring actions by institutions and people.[7]

Given the slackness of Lutheranism in its Icelands, the divided and half-informed Lutheranism in its Detroits and Minnesotas, and the assaults on tradition by modernity, Peterson may be too sanguine. Yet all kinds of resources have to be called upon to promote humaneness and well-being. Those who today live by centuries-old traditions that have survived in many cultures and places may well have much to say about morals and ethics. Not all of it has yet been clearly understood in the culture. Nor is it at hand even among all of those who, within the tradition, claim to have been formed and informed by it.

Part III

PASSAGES

·7·

Sexuality, Family Life, and Generativity

Few aspects of human well-being receive as must attention in the churches, including the Lutheran tradition, as does sexuality. Whereas sex was once a taboo subject and death was discussed openly, today sex is spoken about freely and death is taboo. This once-negative attitude toward sex does not quite hold true in the Christian churches and, more specifically, the Lutheran churches. They have devoted more attention to discussing dimensions of sexual life than almost any other topic in the categories of health, medicine, and physical existence. Sex was not taboo at the time of Lutheran origins, and it receives attention now.

Few aspects of creation determine more of a person's life than sexual differentiation. While unisex fashions have emerged and while male and female roles are drawing closer and overlapping, the differing functions associated with generation and procreation, the differing societal expectations, and the variety of outlooks appropriate or natural to males and females color most other experiences. Out of respect for these differences, all Christian traditions have wrestled with the meaning of sexuality in creation. They have forced much moral and ethical talk. And they have paid sexuality the respect of recognizing that if it is fulfilling and follows plausible norms it can enhance life. Misconstrued, misunderstood, or malpracticed, it can lead to repression, libertinism, and distortion of the rest of life. Sex and well-being are indissolubly linked.

THE USEFULNESS OF THE FAITH TRADITION

As with most elements of health and medicine, the scientific and cultural dimensions of sexuality call for constant adapting in the faith traditions. Even the most conservative Lutherans readily recognize that Luther's and the Bible's views of sexuality are conditioned by the cultural outlook in and during which they first appeared. Whoever goes back to the earliest Lutheran writings for detailed prescriptions for sexual living and health soon finds it impossible to follow them or undesirable even to picture following them. Formal Lutheran writings of two generations ago on such subjects as birth control or divorce sound antique. Their regulations go unenforced; their understandings produce snickers.

Given such gaps between past and present, there may be good reasons to keep the door to the tradition closed, to clamp the lid on the lockbox in which historians guard the antique teachings and counsels. Or shall one open them to produce shudders or shrugs of shoulders, and then close them, curiosities having been gratified? What sense does it make to read them in order to pick and choose what confirms one's present sexual choices and then to reject or ignore those that are inconvenient and embarrassing? Would not an evening be better spent with *The Joy of Sex* or present-day Christian counsel than with a tracing of older Lutheran views?

One answer to such questions is that contemporary Christians should *never* bother with the lore of their lineage. Yet more serious reflection results in a caution. The Lutheran teachings on sexuality are not *only* culturally conditioned. Some do flow out of the center of this church's understanding of faith. To the degree that the center and sexual life are linked, the sexual teachings can either create problems or produce better well-being. Second, in many contexts there are elements of Lutheran teaching that can positively inform sexuality today. Third, getting some sense of changes in Lutheran understandings on this subject can be liberating. To the degree that some Lutherans in the past were damaged by the sexual counsel of their churches, it is liberating for new generations to recognize that not everything once taught by Luther, the orthodox scholars, or pastoral counselors from the past is written in concrete or is to be seen as the law of God.

The greatest change between the present situation and most of the past is the crowding in of the surrounding pluralist culture. Of course, what people around the churches have thought and done has always colored the outlooks of the churches. But in the modern world, mass media of communication—television, cinema, radio, phonograph records, advertising, and the printed page—all present sexual images and counsel that openly contradict what the churches teach. Meanwhile, the churches grow closer to each other. Differences on such matters as sex are often greater within than between traditions. Certain Lutherans link with certain Catholics in affirming body and sex, whereas other Lutherans connect with other Catholics in seeing them negatively. The tradition, therefore, meets competition from without and is blurred from within.

The Lutheran tradition has been very fluid on the sexual theme. One can trace several periods and a succession of attitudes already within the career of Martin Luther. The scholastics who followed him often nailed things down and were far more ordered, strict, and repressive than he. Through the years, Lutheran Pietists and Rationalists have shaped and changed the lore. In our own time the pastoral counsel of Lutheran churches, from the most conservative to the most liberal, has been influenced by therapeutic notions that grew up outside the church and were uninformed by theology. On most substantial sexual topics, one can expect constant fluidity, process, and change. Thoughtful people will also look for some continuities, some basic root values.

LUTHERAN INSIGHTS

The fundamental Lutheran insight into the value of sexuality came early but not instantly. Martin Luther, shaped by a monastic tradition, rejected forced celibacy for priests and helped invent the Protestant parsonage, an important symbol. The marital couple and the family were a strong part of Christian vocational thinking. The God who forgives smiles more on the Christian parents-to-be who are begetting than on the monk who prattles prayers. The sexually tied companionship of a Christian husband and wife may have an equal and, soon, a higher ranking in the sight of God than does the communal life of those in a monastery.

Not all aspects of the monastic tradition and the inherited outlooks disappeared at the same time and with the same force. Monks were taught to have essential'y negative views of the sexual act. It belonged more to the order of sin than to the order of creation. That being the case, Luther and his colleagues had a difficult time giving a truly positive reading to the sexual act. Yet sexuality, linked especially with procreation, was a very positive sign of a loving God's care. Sex was sacred, which is why it was so dangerous, so easily misunderstood or misused.

As Luther developed and after he married, he did not lose his realism about the threatening aspects of sexuality, but he countered these with ever more positive statements about its value. An archaic book on Luther well summarized his mature position on marriage, which was the focus of all sexual expression.

> In the existence of the sexes [Luther] saw the natural basis of marriage, and in revelation he found it a divine institution. The vices of the monks and the Romish clergy exhibited the demoralizing effects of the natural law of celibacy. Hence, both by his example and in his writings, Luther defends what nature and God alike enjoin. . . . Luther says, "Next to God's Word, the world has not a more lovely and endearing treasure on earth than the holy state of matrimony, which He has Himself instituted,

preserving it, having adorned and blessed it above all stations, from which not only all emperors, kings, and saints, but even the eternal Son of God, though in a supernatural way, are born. Whoever, therefore, hates the married state and speaks evil of it, certainly is of the devil."[1]

It was natural that the Reformation began by discussing sexuality and marriage over against the monastic life, since this was near the heart of the Protestant revolt. This issue is by no means central to most Christian lay people's lives today, when monasticism and celibacy are the choice of very few, even very few Catholics. But the battle to elevate marriage beyond celibacy informed whatever has followed in Lutheranism. The monastic vows were to have been forever, yet most of the early Lutheran ministers had been monks who had to break vows. This meant that they had to work out very strong rationales for themselves and the world. In the process, marriage came to be a vehement alternative, to be strenuously defended.

Luther came to urge those who were entering the ministry not to take vows against marriage. If a priest had become involved sexually with a woman, he should turn honest and marry her, no matter what the law, the pope, or the people thought. Since they had sexual relations, in the sight of God they were betrothed, which, in Luther's book, was equivalent to being married in the Christian sense. Why oppose the old vows? Here Lutheran consistency is clear. It is carried over into the view that marriage is not a sacrament. The vows were part of the attempt to impress God, to merit salvation. Yet ties with God should depend upon grace and faith. Not all people are made for celibacy, so how can they promise to be celibate? Luther thought that all are equipped for marriage. Vows in connection with human bonding of couples therefore could be fulfilled.

Luther's outlook called him to condemn the idea of elevating virginity as such to a high status. If one would really spell out its meaning, those who believed the Bible would repudiate their praise of it, and that would be all to the good. To hold back sexual expression, in Luther's eyes, was unnatural, probably impossible. Only people who possessed a rare gift for continence could be expected to follow it. For those who found it unnatural, attempts to remain virginal would lead to terrible desires,—"burning"—and, likely, to sin. Celibacy and virginity, then, might be appreciated in Lutheranism only if they are seen as special gifts and not as something that should impress God.

In his writings, Luther turned again and again to themes that place a high value on marriage and with it, on marital sexual expression. It was God who instituted marriage and made it holy, who induced men and women to fall in love, to seek companionship, to want to express themselves in sexual acts. God had planted drives in our nature, drives that could be used terribly against divine purpose or ecstatically to support that purpose. Already in Eden marriage was present. God saw the creation as good. Two of the Ten Commandments gave support to all that marriage implied.

One cannot, however, collate all of Luther's teachings and see only liter- ally affirmative expression in them. He was generally a Catholic conserva- tive, a schoolman, when it came to discussing the physical side of sex. Sex- ual copulation, though viewed as good inside marriage by 100 percent of polled Lutheran counselors in the twentieth century, was not viewed so positively in Luther's day. It was part of the Fall. So Luther had been taught, and he could not easily or early jump out of the skin that had held him as he learned this. Of course, all that "natural" man and women do, including praying, is "sinful" apart from the grace of God in Christ. But Luther calls special attention to coitus as a blight resulting from the Fall of Adam and Eve. People engrossed in that act in our time may be seen to be living out a holy purpose. For Luther they were sinning, but theirs was a sin for which forgiveness was easy. While copulating, people were not worshiping or praising God. He had been taught to think of sexual expres- sion as unclean, and he thought that his followers would feel the same way during the sexual act.

Almost everyone who writes on Luther's view likes to quote some of his notoriously unflattering passages: "No matter what praise is given to mar- riage, I will not concede it to nature that it is no sin." Because males cannot contain their desires or their semen, they need females, wives, to relate to them in acts that are as natural as drinking and eating—but are somehow more suspect. One marries and continues to sin even in the central physical act of marriage. But one does not then sin as much as were he or she to burn with desire or to find extramarital relief for this burning. Woman, in Lu- ther's view, was a vessel for man, submissive to him, created for creating and bearing a new generation of childbearers and the men who seek relief with them.[2]

So sure was Luther that men would burn with evil desires if unmarried, that he was slightly open to unconventional (for his time) marital arrange- ments. He never knew quite what to make of polygamy or, better, poly- gyny. A devoted student of the Bible, he knew that the holy patriarchs in the Old Testament practiced it without losing the favor of God. He was, however, against the practice in his own time. In a letter, Luther wrote that since "there is no necessity for it, no benefits in it, and no special word of God commanding it," it should not be practiced. But he also could find no divine commandment against it. In extreme cases, it might be possible

that a person must go "beyond the liberty which is conditioned by love."
We have seen that he counseled bigamy in at least one instance.[3]

In the end, Luther came back to monogamy: "Marriage is an eternal
and orderly joining together of one man and one woman. I say, the union
of *one* man and *one* woman, not many, because God says that two shall be
one flesh. For a man to have several wives is against the natural law."

Curiously, Luther finally condemned polygyny more on the grounds
that it did not meet present-day custom than that it opposed the Word of
God. Christ was for monogamy only, but

> Abraham did not commit adultery by leading a decent life with his second
> wife also. Abraham was a true Christian. His example dare not be con-
> demned. It is true, one dare not make any laws out of the behavior of our
> forefathers, but one may not make sin out of their example.[4]

All that can be made of this whole dimension of Reformation teaching is
that adultery was so evil that bigamy or polygymy were to be preferred.
There is not much to go on here for our contemporaries.

Luther's great change came in 1520. He determined then that marriage
was not a sacrament, since it did not convey grace. God, however, did institute and bless it, and sexuality came along within marriage. The only
way to make sexuality and marriage holy was to listen to how God saved
couples, through the good news of forgiveness in Christ. There will be sins
particularly in sexual expression in marriage, but one should fight off lust
and ask for forgiveness, which God is ready and eager to give. God com-
manded marriage. God placed sexual desire in people and provided this
marital way for gratifying it. Married people could not deny sex to each
other. To do so was a form of adultery, which could lead legitimately to divorce. In the Bible, King Ahasuerus legitimately left Vashti for a more com-
pliant Esther after some warnings. Luther, blinded by his male vision, argued that men in his time could do the same. With typical boisterousness he
solved the problem: "If the wife refuse, let the maid come!"—a counsel
more radical than what one is likely to hear from a Lutheran adviser today.

In the early Lutheran view, God is seen as the neighbor, as the hidden
Christ—especially in the spouse. When spouses love each other, they are
being Christs to each other. Whenever they come together, couples should
remember the Fall. Whenever they come together, they also should rejoice
in union because of the forgiveness God has given. Since there was so much
theological meaning in sex, people should talk about it. Luther, a plain-
spoken person, resented prudishness or any taboo on the subject. People
would feel shame if sex were to be a hush-hush subject. He was all for the

sex education of the young. Whoever finds sex too shameful or intimate a topic for discussion cannot appeal to the roots of the Lutheran tradition.[5]

In the matter of sex and marriage, the Lutheran tradition makes much of Luther, whose own struggles did so much to help invent the tradition. Thus the power of sex in human life becomes clear from Luther's confessions about his monastic years. Sexual drives were not central to his concept of the sins he did not feel were forgiven. They were not the focus of leaving his monastery. Yet he was honest enough to pay sex the compliment of recognizing its thrall:

> When I was a monk I thought that I was utterly damned if at any time I felt the concupiscence of the flesh; that is to say, if I felt any evil motive, fleshly lust [*libidenem*], wrath, hatred, or envy against my brother. I tried many ways, I went to confession daily, etc., but nothing helped; for the concupiscence of my flesh always returned so that I could not rest.
>
> I was a chaste monk as a young man but I also felt my old Adam at work.... When a young man sees a pretty girl he lusts after her even against his own will.
>
> As a monk I did not feel great sexual desire, I had [nocturnal] pollutions which were expressions of bodily impulses.

The struggle was not easy, but there is every reason to believe Luther when he says that he was premaritally chaste. Yet, "I have been a monk and have given up sleep, fasted, prayed, castigated and tormented my body, all in order to maintain obedience and chastity." It is not necessary to picture all subsequent Lutherans having to be so hard on themselves as was this ex-monk. Thus marriage is not necessarily such a great contrast to a previous way of life. Like so many other Christians throughout history, Luther "thought that there was no greater sin on earth than unchastity." Yet, because he was poised between doubt and faith, the spiritual temptations he thought God sent were more plaguing to Luther than were the physical temptations the devil sent.

THE ISSUE OF MARRIAGE

Luther began to sever ties with Rome in 1517 and married eight years later, hardly a short time had the desire for marriage been strong. He wed ex-nun Katherine von Bora a bit reluctantly. Throughout his life he chronicled the ups and downs of this marriage in memorable phrases, most of which we shall have to resist the temptation to quote. He saw Katie working to make him a fixed star while he was an irregular planet. Yet she succeeded in ordering much of his life, whereas he tried to dominate her.

His home life became a model for later Protestant parsonages. Katie found ways to instruct him. His compliments were not always of the highest order:

> I would not trade my Katie for France or Venice for three reasons: first, because God gave her to me as a gift and also gave me to her; second, because I often come across other women with far more shortcomings than Katie, and although she has a few weaknesses of her own, they are far outnumbered by her virtues; and third, because faith serves marriage best through its fidelity and honor.

Marriage for Luther was a civil act, not chiefly a concern of the church. On regulating marriage, he wrote, "The pope has as little power to command this, as he had to forbid eating, drinking, the natural movement of the bowels, or growing fat."[6] In these respects, marriage was curiously secular and clearly nonsacramental. Each civil province could find different laws for marriage. "Surely no one can deny that marriage is an external, a secular affair, subject to secular government, as are clothing and food, house and home." Christ and the apostles did not concern themselves with marital regulation. The whole endeavor has to be seen in light of human law and natural law:

> To forbid marriage is contrary to nature. How can you forbid and condemn marriage, which is one of the natural rights? You do not forbid a man to eat, drink, and sleep, do you? What God has made and ordered does not stand in our choice. We dare not take it or forbid it.

The Lutheran tradition comes to a formal center in sixteenth-century creedal confessions. They have little to say on the subject of sex and marriage. They oppose secret engagements carried on beyond parental view, hardly a controverted point today. More positively, and here let me quote a collation by modern scholars of quotations from Article XXIII of the Apology of the Augsburg Confession:

> Gen. 1:28 teaches that men were created to be fruitful and that one sex in a proper way should desire the other . . . This [physical] love of one sex for the other is truly a divine ordinance. . . . Just as by human laws the nature of the earth cannot be changed, so, without a special work of God, the nature of a human being can be changed neither by vows nor by human law. . . . Since natural right is immutable, the right to contract marriage must always remain. . . . They [the Roman Catholics] proclaim that they require celibacy because it is purity. As though marriage were impurity and a sin, or as though celibacy merited justification more than does marriage. . . . [Marriage] is a pure, holy, noble, praiseworthy work of God.

That is not much to go on, even with the addition of a few other fugitive lines such as this one from the Apology of the Augsburg Confession: "Marriage is *jus naturale*, and as factual existence it holds a divine mandate and divine promise."

These limited views have been elaborated on by most modern Lutheran churches. Typical of the much more positive extension is a statement by the old United Lutheran Church in America at a turning point, in 1956. The marriage union is in the Christian view the joining

> of a man and a woman in a one-flesh relation which is a mystery like the union of Christ and His church. The basis of this union was laid when God created man in His own image and "made them male and female." Thus, man and woman were made to complement and enrich each other in a purposeful and covenanted relation.... Love, as agape, seeks to know and serve the other's needs, driving one out of the "I" into relation with the "Thou." This encounter should bear witness to and foretell the richness of man's encounter with God in Christ.

One glance will show that the modern statements of this sort are more congruent with biblical views of sexuality and marriage than were the early Lutheran ones, conditioned as these were by a millennium of more negative views in Catholicism.

When modern Lutherans remain negative, one of their own will chide them. Thus in the face of negative comment, theologian Martin J. Heinecken in 1957 complained of "a deep-seated malady, something gone wrong with the basic orientation toward sex." It was "high time that the church cease lamenting and denouncing and give a theological diagnosis and suggest a theological cure, in positive, constructive terms." Otherwise people would fall into mere sensuality and seek "the frantic multiplication of piecemeal satisfactions because the quality of life has lost its eternity."[7] Such whipping into action contrasts favorably with ancient Lutheran crabbiness in the scholastic period, when there was more passivity and bemoaning of the world.

By the time Heinecken was writing, other Lutherans were taking up the challenge of presenting a positive view. Harold Haas, writing for the United Lutheran Church, was emphatic in setting a new tone, in helping see the new direction in Lutheran understanding of sex and well-being. It included an implied scolding of Luther and other foreparents:

> When the sexual union is thought of either as something intrinsically evil or simply as a biological outlet, then marriage can at best serve only a remedy against sin, a socially sanctioned control of an instinct, or an unwarranted bond interfering with individual freedom.

> Sexual union has, however, a far more profound meaning than either of
> these alternatives. The creation which God declared to be good contained
> within it the physical encounter of sex between man and woman. It is true
> that the sinful condition of man can be expressed through sex in a pro-
> found and far-reaching way. This does not alter the basic fact, however,
> that sex as given by God is good.

The tradition develops consistently with its biblical genius, even if it must
repudiate some of its own Lutheran ancestry. The view psychologist Haas
expresses for a modern church body is certainly more congruent with Lutheran understandings of the body than are the narrow, cramping, early
postcelibate understandings of Luther and the confessions.[8]

MALE AND FEMALE
AND THE PASSAGE OF TIME

The roots of the Lutheran tradition are problematic as far as male and
female roles are concerned. Lutheran culture may not have devoted itself so
systematically to expression of sexual *macho* as some Latin cultures have. In
cultural and domestic expression, however, it can rightfully be accused of
stretching male dominance far beyond what is implied in biblical texts.

The early writers built on Saint Paul's teachings about the priority and
dominance of Adam in the creation. Similarly, the impetus was thence given
for subordinate and submissive attitudes on the part of women. *Kinder, Kir-
che, Küche*—children, church, kitchen—were stressed so strongly that the
roles became proverbial on German Lutheran soil. Women and men today
struggle to understand sexual roles while extricating the core of their traditions from the cultural accretions of Germany, Scandinavia, or America in
centuries past.

The limits of Lutheran teaching, the exaggerations of biblical talk about
male priority, and Lutheran patriarchalism are qualified somewhat from
the first, however, by the strong accents on companionship, mutuality,
and regard for both spouses' desires and needs within a consummated marriage.

To illustrate the power of culture to reshape even a conservative tradition such as Lutheranism in matters of sex and marriage it is worthwhile
noting the virtual disappearance of old Lutheran teaching on the meaning
of engagement. The issue was still controverted at mid-century by a conservative Lutheran group, the Missouri Synod. As a result, we have excellent studies of twentieth-century attitudes by Lutherans on this subject.
Few Lutherans in the 1980s would argue that spiritually betrothal is "tan-
tamount" to marriage. Luther, historic Lutheranism, and modern Mis-

sourians did so. To make sense of the raging controversy, the Missourians took a poll of families in three Lutheran synods. Almost half of the Missouri Synod families and 69 percent of the clergy considered engagement to be marriage in the sight of God; the percentages were much lower in other synods.

Luther, relying also on Old Testament passages, inherited from the Middle Ages the idea that betrothal was much the same as marriage. He could consider the breaking of an engagement to be less, but only slightly less, sinful than a divorce apart from the cause of adultery. "Whoso touches another with betrothal after the public betrothal, so as to marry her, to break the first betrothal, that should be regarded as adultery."

It is clear that Luther associated conjugal rights with betrothal, and thus saw marriage as a mere civil act. Luther wanted engagements to be brief; why not engagement, civil marriage, and coital consummation the same night? Dogmatic Lutherans later thought that one kind of engagement could not be dissolved. It was unconditional. They began, however, to stress the role of the marital promise as the time when marriage began. "I do *now* take thee as wife." Almost 40 percent of Missouri Synod members believed that conjugal privileges should go with engagement. For a time that church body made its engagement views a matter to help divide the synod from other Lutheran bodies. To break an engagement could mean excommunication.

All that is changed today. Here is a case where scholarly study led to change and correction within a tradition. The surrounding culture clearly did not assign the old Hebrew scriptural status to betrothal. The understanding of the act had shifted. So the conservative Lutheran body, after exploring the tradition, also shifted. It grew emphatic that engaged people should stop having sex with each other simply on the grounds that in the Hebrew Scriptures betrothal provided that license. Meanwhile, it stopped enacting stern discipline in the case of those who broke engagements. The whole teaching that once agitated a church, divided it from other Lutherans, and produced immense trauma in the lives of individuals has become a curiosity, is unrecognized by the younger generation, has almost slipped from view. Traditions can correct themselves in light of their genius.[9]

CHANGES IN CONCEPTS OF
BIRTH CONTROL AND AUTOEROTICISM

For another example of change, one might consult almost any popular Lutheran pastoral manual of a half century ago to read a consistent and universal criticism of "artificial" birth control. A few decades later almost all Lutherans were advocating family planning, all in the interest of stewardship, with the use of many kinds of devices. Among conservative Lutherans a best seller was Walter A. Maier's, *For Better Not for Worse*. Maier was an immensely popular radio preacher, perhaps the best-known American Lutheran of his time. His was a book-length attack on birth control.

It is not necessary to read all of Maier; his chapter titles reveal the viewpoint of this representative Lutheran leader: "The Blight of Birth Control," "An Outrage against Nature," "A Moral Degradation," "A Divorce Stimulus," "A Menace to National Prosperity," "Crafty Commercialism," "Its Anti-Scriptural Bias." Maier attacked modern churches for being for birth control—yet they held positions his own church allowed and encouraged a decade or two later. "The Church must maintain [that if having children] is evaded . . . through the employment of methods suggested by birth control, divine displeasure is invoked." Only three lines in a fifty-page chapter refer to licit "natural" methods. "The Church has never protested against the employment of those means which the course of nature itself seems to provide, unless their employment is a selfish attempt to evade the responsibilities of parenthood." Maier could still boast that "the Lutheran Church is definitely arrayed against birth restriction."[10]

I bring this up not to sneer at the recent past or to cast doubt upon the tradition so much as to say that on decisive matters the tradition has been fluid. Something of a higher value such as conjugality, companionship, and stewardship, in combination, can replace firm notions based on more simple legalism or cultural reactionism. No one need claim that the more modern period always brings more enlightenment. Certainly some old sexual codes and practices produced more good than do some more modern codes or therapies. But health and medicine matters remain in flux and demand constant reappraisal.

The Lutheran tradition has apparently also moderated on autoerotic practices. A conservative American tract from around the period of World War I saw masturbation to be "a heathen vice," "undermining body and soul and ruining health," "stunting growth," and converting a person into a "liar whose lying is second nature." Many become insane, it was charged, because of "self-abuse." "The law condemns everyone who carnally knows himself [sic] or a brute or another person of the same sex."[11]

More recent American Lutheranism would not put a premium on masturbation or even clearly approve it. It has, however, dropped from the list of prime sins. The cultural superstitions concerning its consequences are no longer associated with it. By 1959 William E. Hulme of the American Lutheran Church was seeing masturbation as an escape from reality and an unnecessary inducer of guilt, but he made less of it.[12]

COITION AND THE END OF MARRIAGE

In the Lutheran tradition it is clear that coital expression has been limited to marriage after the concept of equating betrothal to marriage fell out of favor. Extramarital sex, because it violates a promise and exercises infidelity, receives the more vehement criticism. Premarital sex is also frowned upon. Through the years, however, it is clear that the Lutheran concept of the gospel has led its pastors and counselors to place sexual sins in a somewhat different light than formerly. Without minimizing the importance of deviation from the marital norm, the modern manuals stress that sexual sins are by no means necessarily so socially disruptive as, say, racial prejudice or social injustices. And although one is consistently critical of the lapse, there is room for continued acceptance of the lapsed one. Most of these topics, however, have to do more with moral fault than with physical well-being.

The same is true of divorce; it is seen more as a moral issue than one that directly affects the physical well-being of the individual. At the same time, counselors in this tradition recognize that disruption of obedience to a law of God or acceptance of a way of life the individual recognizes to be incongruent with the revealed divine will can well lead to guilt. For Luther, adultery was not a grounds for divorce; it *was* a divorce. The sinned-against partner was urged to grant forgiveness, but in a sense a divorce had already occurred.

Through the years Luther moved from wanting the death penalty for adulterers who caused divorce to merely commenting on the spiritual death of the adulterer. The aggrieved partner was free to remarry. It is hard to find a pattern in Luther's view of divorce; he seems to have been arbitrary and erratic in his approvals and disapprovals. He set the historic precedent for Lutheran disapproval of divorce and pastoral reconstruction of the lives of the divorced. In his vocabulary, however, such words as *incompatibility* did not yet play a part. Nor, in the Lutheran confessions, did religious "mixed marriage" and its tensions legitimate divorce.[13]

A modern study of Luther by William M. Lazareth concentrates on the pastoral counseling of Luther, especially in matters of divorce. He savagely criticized the Catholic counsel, speaking of one book as something "whose contents have been poured together out of the cesspool of all human traditions." Thus, when there has been some marital problem, the priests force an errant man to remain in his wife's bed but not to have intercourse with her. "They put dry wood on the fire and say, Do not burn. They put a man in a woman's arms and forbid him to touch her or know her. And they do this on their own authority and without the command of God. What madness?" Luther wanted more realism.

Here Luther ranked the keeping of marital vows higher than taking monastic ones. A man might acquire a dissolution of marital vows in order to join a religious order. "The pope decrees that a marriage is dissolved if one partner enters a monastery even without the consent of the other, provided the marriage be not yet consummated. O what devil puts such monstrous things into the pope's mind!"

Lazareth finds great fault with Luther's counsel. His motivation was pastoral. Luther wanted to offer forgiveness, but his field was limited by the legal situation. "Nevertheless, the content of Luther's early marital counsel, whatever the motivation and the circumstances, is naive at best and illegal at worst." Thus, as we have seen, when Philip of Hesse could not contain himself sexually inside an arranged marriage, Luther counseled him to be a bigamist and to lie when charged with bigamy. In these and similar cases he revealed his limits. But he also seemed to know them, and in one case said, "Herewith I hang up my harp, until another and a better man shall take up this matter with me." Many a latter-day Lutheran has wished Luther would have hung up his harp sooner.[14]

·8·

The Passages of Life, the Phases of Faith

The search for well-being and the understandings of health and medicine changes their character for all persons as they pass through the various developmental stages of life. The senior citizen in the nursing home may be involved in a round-the-clock preoccupation with buttoning and unbuttoning, taking pills and temperatures, giving advice and seeking counsel, fearing death and facing death. He can hardly recall the day when he was once an All-American football tackle whose physical pains were only the result of bruised ankles. The young child afflicted with a conquerable disease of infancy is dependent on others for being well. Her needs have little in common with those problems she will have at the onset of puberty or in her own childbearing years. Just as religious traditions, even though they have continuity, are not constant, so each human life is a "tradition." This means that it is a handing over of a genetic package and a set of possibilities within an always and also ever-changing person.

Religion has always recognized the stages of life. Childhood, we have heard, was "invented" or discovered not many centuries ago. Before this, children were regarded sartorially and behaviorally as miniature adults. The church Catholic had already by then devised elaborate rites of infant initiation. These recognized special needs. Before modern developmental psychologists elaborated theories on adolescence, Jewish and Christian ceremonies of education and ritual helped mark changes in phases of personal life. The medical study of aging is a modern invention, yet ancient scriptures already concerned themselves with understanding how people should face the decline of physical life and the completion of personal being.

Not all and not even most religious traditions have concerned themselves with specific medical applications to all these changing scripts in the life of each human. There is no Baptist potion for infants, Buddhist lotion for adolescents, Muslim herb for people at mid-life, or Lutheran pharmaceutical prescription for the aged.

Informed people in each tradition work at the side of medical professionals to help assure that, in the division of human labor, appropriate scientific research and application both go on. Here, for Lutherans, the doctrine of the calling or vocation has an important bearing. This honors the laboratory technician and the psychiatrist as they go about their special work. There is little religious "stepping in" with medical counsel in all their work. Even wholistic religious understandings recognize some division of labor. Those who hold to them may possess no special grasp of test tubes or CAT scans. They bring something else from their sides of the division of labor.

RELIGIOUS RITES AND
INTERPRETATIONS OF PASSAGE

Not surprisingly, the gifts of religious traditions have to do with prayers appropriate to each age. They reveal theological ponderings of what each period in life unfolds. Traditions include appropriate kinds of counsel and care, urging believers to "be with" others. Finally, or first of all, there are rites of passage. Long before *Passages* by Gail Sheehy became a best seller, long before Lawrence Kohlberg outlined stages of moral development or Erik Erikson discerned and expounded a sequence of "crises" in life as people sought identities, and long before these rites had a name, ceremonies of passage characterized most religions. Included among these is the Lutheran branch of the Christian Church.

European Lutheranism owns up to some rueful jokes about at least three of these. Some cynics speak of them as exemplifying "four-wheel" Christianity. People who are otherwise not involved come to the house of God at least three times on four wheels: in the carriage for infant baptism, the limousine for marriage, and the hearse for burial. Another phrase has it that people need the church at least for ceremonies that go along with being "hatched, matched, and dispatched."

The phrases and jokes disguise a deep hurt. The church stands ready to do more for people's well-being. It can be of far more help than standing by with a handful of baptismal water, a priestly stole to wrap around wedding rings during a blessing, or a little bit of reading from a black book to go with the earth thrown upon a coffin. The church increasingly wishes to provide understandings of the distinctive issues of health and medicine that medical specialists are addressing in other ways.

In profound traditions, rites are never "mere" rites. When people say, "Oh, that was just a lot of ceremony," or "It was only the liturgy," they fail to understand what sacraments and ritual have meant or are intended to mean in such faith lineages. Rites have a certain kind of therapeutic role.

This is most evident if we keep in mind the fact that over the ages religion has been an instrument for social bonding. It helps provide security to members of a group. Of course, negatively, it may also become an instrument of repression when it threatens people with becoming outsiders to a group. This can be a very high price to pay. Positively, rites help people relate "I" to "Thou," time to eternity, generations to each other, persons to environments. Each of these relations has an obvious bearing on mental, spiritual, and often even physical well-being.

Two generations of sociologists have defined religion as a system of beliefs and practices by which people try to make sense of a universe. "Because we are present to a world, we are condemned to meaning," says philosopher Maurice Merleau-Ponty.[1] The search for meaning pushes unprepared individuals into unfamiliar situations and places them on threatening horizons. Rites help make the passages easier, even satisfying. Lloyd Warner observed American communities and located them right alongside primitive religion: "All societies ritualize and publicly mark with suitable observances to impress the significance of the individual and the group on living members of the community. These are the important times of birth, puberty, marriage and death."

The acts associated with being born and dying are the great traumas or crises of all life. Before birth the fetus seems more of an "It" than a "Thou." At once, after birth "It" takes on personal characteristics and comes to be loved in new ways. Similarly, death is seen by most people as a passage toward unsorted, unspecified forms of existence. Despite centuries of secularization and deritualization, however, death still calls forth some efforts at ritualization from even the most complex societies. In the understanding of the passages of life, the individual joins a larger world. The larger concepts of the world then get applied to the life of the individual.

Victor Turner, a recent student of ritual passages, quoted Arnold van Gennep, the inventor of the modern concept of *rites de passage*, in order to define three aspects or processes in each case. A stage of separation (*separation*) passes through one of transition (*marge*) to a third, of incorporation (*agrégation*). In the first phase, the individual is set aside, cut off from the group. Then follows a "betwixt and between stage," as Turner calls it, while a person passes over a threshold, a *limen*. After this she is reincorporated into the group, but now on a new level. All "rights and privileges attendant thereto" in the new context now support the individual.[2]

These rites have a bearing far beyond what goes on within the walls of the church. Wholistic health experts are connecting them, and the understandings that go with them, with developmental stages in both the physical body and the psychic outlook of individuals. Each concept calls forth somewhat different grasps of what character and responsibility are, or what demands morals and ethics make upon the person in the new stage. This is another reason why different religious traditions have somewhat different words for those who seek well-being. They depend in part upon where in their life stages believers find themselves. Each new medical possibility also imposes a demand for new ethical understandings.

The modern focus upon the prenatal stages of the first passage, the transit from fetal life to personhood as a child, is the most debated today. The Lutheran literature, up until a generation or two ago, was very sparse. Although there was always some talk about birth control, no one foresaw genetic experimentation, artificial insemination, *in vitro* fertilization, or the complexity of the modern abortion debates. So many laboratory discoveries have occurred within a mere decade that experts in bioethics can concern themselves with these issues over the length of a career and not begin to exhaust their ethical implications.

Here we must resist the temptation to turn this book into a technical essay on bioethics. We have determinedly understood it as a general book on the search for being well, a comment on meanings out of which ethics emerges. Now and then Lutheran church bodies have made statements on the issues of conception and prenatal life, particularly in the case of abortion. They have on occasion sponsored medical and theological seminars on such subjects. Here and there a Lutheran bioethicist of note has written on some complex aspects of one of these subjects. In all instances, there have been conscious and unconscious efforts to draw upon the tradition. The tradition, however, could hardly have presented much explicit teaching, since there was little of a technical character about which to teach.

CONCEPTION AND WHAT FOLLOWS

Through four centuries Lutheranism had only a few clear things to say about conception. It should occur between married people. It calls forth demands for responsibility. There is a call for care for both the mother and the fetus. People must rearrange life to care for the eventually emergent child. The mother, it was assumed, had prime concern for care, but the father was to be at her side. Necessarily, on theological terms, a full Christian marriage included an obligation to procreate. God intended marriage to this end. To refuse to help create a new generation violated the law of God. Lutherans should practice sexual restraint or follow women's natural cycles if they wished to plan their parenthood and limit the number of children. If a fetus aborted through miscarriage, it was simply disposed of. There was no recognition of personhood, no sign of individuality of the sort Lutherans associate with infant baptism, though, if there was a possibility of life in the "stillborn," there would be an emergency baptism. That was that. There was little more, nor did there then need to be.

From the time of Luther on, the tradition treated the problem of impotence, which could be a cause for the annulment of a marriage. Similarly, a complete refusal by a partner to consummate a marriage or to participate in sexual activity was a denial of the biblical view of marriage and effectively barred the possibility of procreation. Thus the practice was also a denial of the integrity of marriage and grounds for divorce.

What if the couple cooperated in sexual activity and yet there was no conception? Lutheran counsel would then urge adoption of an orphan so there could be a family. Then it had to fall silent, as did all other counsel in a time when people knew nothing of conception science. Perhaps folk piety and superstition might evoke calls for the use of the mandrake root or some other stimulant to conception. There was apparently little opposition to fertility drugs as these developed, though ethicists have always cautioned about the medical risks involved with them. The Lutheran tradition could not have had much more to do or to say until the genetic breakthroughs of the late twentieth century.

If one may risk a generalization about informed Lutheran bioethicists: they tend to find congenial the counsel of the more conservative ethicists such as Paul Ramsey. Such people urge the policy of "going slowly," when in doubt, on subjects like *in vitro* fertilization ("test-tube babies"). There is some concern over "playing God," and more fear lest something might possibly go wrong. People may generate genetic accidents instead of people. Or there may be unforeseen psychological problems for parents and child after the fetus is conceived in a test tube. "Go slow" does not, however, mean "go not at all."

Lacking panels of ethicists on the subject, I asked Bishop David Preus, an experienced pastor and president of the American Lutheran Church, about his impression on "test-tube babies" in the context of his church. Would a Lutheran hospital that bears the name "American Lutheran" feel strictures against such experimentation and achievement? Preus began his answer with all of the "go slow" cautions that are so becoming within the Lutheran tradition. Yet in the end, after all the cautions and reservations, he thought Lutheranism would not discourage and would even quietly encourage efforts made to have those who could not conceive otherwise do so through these means. The theologians he consulted and respected agreed that Lutheranism puts extreme emphasis on the family. It is so understanding of maternal and paternal drives and on the value of procreation that it would certainly not a priori stand in the way of such endeavors. Preus's view is probably a good summary of mainstream emergent Lutheran ethical positions, but it is too early to elaborate on this.

LUTHERAN DEBATES ON ABORTION

Calm, cool, collected "maybes" and "perhaps" are not likely to fall from the lips of a church president who is interviewed about the debate in his church body over a possible event in the next stage of fetal life. I refer to the issue of abortion in the Lutheran tradition. This issue is far and away the most controversial of all having to do with health and medicine in our decades. It divides denominations, movements, political parties, and living room gatherings. People who ordinarily act very rationally toward each other find themselves drawing on visceral depths and shouting "murderer" or "repressor" across a panel or a crowded room at old and soon-to-be former friends.

Although one cannot say that the abortion debate has taken up many pages in earlier Lutheran theological or ethical thought, the issue has been present. It antedates Lutheranism and Christianity. Is the fetus human? What is it? What are its rights? Since Lutherans have never baptized naturally aborted fetuses, they have evidently not regarded them the way they regarded prematurely born infants. A scan of the contemporary literature suggests that along with most of the Christian tradition, Lutheranism has regarded the life of the mother more highly than that of a fetus. Therefore, if abortion is an almost certain maternal lifesaver at the expense of fetal life, Lutheran ethicists and physicians have generally permitted such therapeutic abortions. This means that they are not usually absolutists about the integrity of fetal rights. The fetus has rights, but the fetus alone does not have all the rights in this tradition. One can read the whole Catholic and Lutheran literature on abortion until it became a political issue in the United States in the 1970s and not see people needing to reach for the word *murderer* to stigmatize those who for various reasons have had abortions or performed them. The emotional and political stage is new.

Whether through involuntary or voluntary means, abortion terminates a pregnancy before a fetus is viable. In the involuntary case the Lutheran simply consigns all to the will and providence of God. A birth was not intended. One reads little into the death of the fetus. The voluntary abortion raises all the theological questions of the beginnings of life and responsibility for its duration, care, and possible termination.

The Lutheran tradition of medical understandings always begins with the Bible, which, unfortunately for those who would simply settle the debate, has only one explicit text (Exod. 21:22–25) on abortion. There was a penalty in Mosaic law on anyone who was guilty of an abortion by accident, as when fighting men hurt a pregnant woman and she aborted. Many scholars read this passage as one that does not express primacy for the fetus as a human being.

The New Testament has nothing to say on the subject. Opponents of abortion read certain biblical passages that refer to "me" after conception as settling the issue of viability, human personality, and rights. From conception, one is a full person, they say, and to take fetal life through abortion is morally the same as taking potent and developed human life. The conservative Lutheran Reformation took over much of the inherited Catholic view of the fetus and of abortion. This meant a general and consistent opposition to the practice.

George Williams, a Unitarian historian at Harvard, has argued that the early reformers, Luther among them, intensified the Catholic position. At least unwittingly, they helped provide the attitudes that led modern popes to condemn abortion more vigorously than did their pre-Reformation predecessors. In their view, from conception on, there was a full human being. Later Lutherans do not or would not have to accept this view at all if later scientific discovery would settle the issue. Unfortunately, it has not and perhaps never can. The debate is likely to remain philosophical and theological. What do you *mean* by life, human life, full human life, personality, and rights? These are questions not settled in the test tube or the laboratory.

Why did Luther and his colleague Melanchthon devote some attention to this medical question? They were inexpert on the subject and not often preoccupied with issues of that type. The two were not preparing themselves for marital counseling or abortion debates. Their concern was with the intense theological questions of original sin, the transmission of guilt from parents to children, the foreknowledge and predestining activity of God. Because they professed a wholistic view of the Fall, which meant that body and soul, physical organism and spirit, were involved, they found it valid to see conception as the "package deal," the "prefabricating moment" that determined what a human being was and was to be. Those terms, obviously, are mine and not theirs. For Luther this meant siding with the ancient traducianists, those who believed that the parents passed on soul and body. The woman was a "vessel." She was the nurturing conduit, whereas the male semen transmitted the life from the originally guilty Adam to the fetus and, hence, the child. Melanchthon, on the other hand, sided with creationists: God made a fresh soul at the instant of conception. But the divine activity at this point in both cases also granted human rights to the fetus. The medical knowledge of the reformers may have been meager, but their theological point, arising on independent grounds, was forceful.[3]

Although the two may not have known much about viability, they did know that they were against abortion as a thwarting of divine purpose for the conceived, potentially full human being at any time. They did not even make Catholic distinctions between the more serious form of abortion for a "formed" fetus and a less serious one for an "unformed" one. The reformers stood only at the beginning of the Lutheran tradition, but their words have to be taken seriously by all sides in debates about abortion.

There would be few abortion debates if Lutherans were literalists about the beginnings of their tradition. They are not. They ignore or find irrelevant or even repulsive many ethical viewpoints of a Luther or a Melanchthon. Open as Lutherans have been to later scientific discovery, they have also been ready to adopt their theological views. Thus their original massive assault on what Catholics call "artificial birth control," a stand that lived on into the middle of the twentieth century in American conservative Lutheranism, disappeared almost without a trace a mere two decades later. It is theoretically possible that new medical knowledge about the fetus could occasion such a change again. We have suggested, however, that practically it is not likely that science will ever satisfyingly decide the issue of what is human life and what rights accompany such understandings.

There would also be no abortion debate if Lutherans were absolutists about the biblical tradition, which they are not. That is, they do not take a single passage in isolation and work out an entire ethical system on the basis of it. The Bible prohibits divorce on more grounds than most Lutherans, including Luther—who abhorred divorce—do or did. There are passages in the gospels that quote Jesus against the taking of life. Pacifists easily use these as absolute prohibitions. Yet, in the main, Lutherans have been militant in war, ready for capital punishment, and defenders of law and order even when it takes the lives of innocents in repressive regimes. One set of values may rule out an absolutist application of others. The issue with abortion is: are there compensatory values strong enough to rule out the Lutheran tradition's strictures against abortion?

Ask conservative Lutheran antiabortionists, "Is abortion murder?" and they may answer after the debates of today in a political time, yes. Ask the same person, "Is there any possibility that you might assent to a therapeutic abortion when the life of the mother almost certainly can be saved at the expense of the fetus or almost certainly will be lost if no effort at abortion is made?" and the answer will almost certainly be yes. This means that the Lutheran is being consistent with the tradition and yet not being an absolutist. In effect, the terms of the debate have then shifted to the more congenial side of historic Lutheranism. The slogan cannot be: "A woman's body is her own to do with what she wants." That is an almost inconceivable way of putting a Lutheran position about responsibility and choice. Nor will "abortion is murder" suffice. That is not a fully accurate rendition of the tradition. It is certainly not a stimulus to fresh inquiry, dialogue, or potential new understanding. Now the proposition might be: "The fetus has rights, but the fetus alone does not have all the rights."

Furthermore, the presence of a debate *within* Lutheranism derives from still another compensatory set of values in the tradition. Life is lived under the cross, in a world of contradiction, paradox, dilemma, ambiguity, and conflict between bad choices. Where there has been fault, there are both judgment and pastoral counsel for restoration of wholeness before God. The tradition foresees action in penitence and contrition, life lived with a stinging conscience and then reenlivened by grace.

Although Lutherans often may forget this, their ethos for the soldier is not one that permits glorying in battle and victory. Fighting is done also "under the cross." With an alert and quickened conscience and the constant need for repentance and grace, the military person acts. After all, the aim of the soldier is to kill another redeemed child of God, perhaps to shorten the period of redemption of that person, to cut off the possibility of his "being saved." This concept should remove the act from its bitter impersonality and make it a terrifying assault on conscience and threat to Christian love. Yet one may have to do such killing. There are theoretical circumstances in which it could be part of a "just" war. Almost all Lutherans no matter what their nations, including Nazi Germany, have felt their wars were just.

Some schools of Lutheranism have similarly treated the subject of abortion. They have reckoned that, in the case of rape or incest, the psychological trauma may be so severe that one may propose the abortion of a nonviable fetus. Or they may determine that, through scientific means unknown to a Luther or a Melanchthon, we may now recognize that a fetus may be doomed to almost subhuman levels of subsequent mental shortcomings. The consistent antiabortionist says that in such cases God is trying to say something to the parents of such potential offspring and may be calling them to a life of meaningful suffering, but others will say that if the fetus comes to full term, the potential is also great for the destruction of meaning in all the lives that surround such a person. Some Lutherans even go so far as to say that the circumstances of a mother may be so psychologically traumatic and physically threatening that she should have some choice about whether or not to carry the fetus to viable status. In general this position has found less support because Lutheranism has been located in places in the culture where these problems have not been too evident and where there are compensatory alternatives, such as adoption of unwanted children.

A fourth occasion for a debate within Lutheranism has had to do with the question of how one opposes abortion. Is it an issue of conscience to people in believing traditions? Should they merely do what they can to convince their own not to have abortions? Or is it an expression of an absolute, something that needs to be forbidden by any humane society just as it must punish murderers? If the former is the case, bearers of the Lutheran tradition have plenty of homework. I have seen computer print-outs from abortion clinics where the religious identifications are linked and have talked to people in the abortion circles who confirm this: the women who are having abortions tend to replicate exactly the religious makeup of the local population. If that population is 30 percent Catholic, 4 percent Jewish, 8 percent Lutheran, 12 percent Baptist, then the percentage of abortion seekers is 30 percent Catholic, 4 percent Jewish, 8 percent Lutheran, 12 percent Baptist. We need social scientific surveys to confirm or disprove such findings. But it is clear that the antiabortion traditions do, in any case, have a great deal of homework. They often are striking out to effect through legislation what they are not succeeding in convincing their own daughters about. Some other Lutherans have argued that if society and the church lack convincing power and rely on legal force alone, this will mean an ineffective and unhealthful resolution. It would be much like Prohibition but with devastating personal consequences.

What I have tried to do in these four or five themes is to show how and why Christian people of Lutheran confession and conscience could divide over the question. That there is division is clear from the fact that some major Lutheran church bodies in denominational conventions have produced somewhat ambiguous statements on abortion. These allow for circumstances of "choice." Similarly, opinion surveys show that although the majority of Lutherans, along with the majority of the population, oppose abortion, they do not favor constitutional amendments prohibiting them. The Lutheran case is complex.

The Lutheran antiabortion forces have been influenced by non-Lutheran conservative politics and ecumenical Christian voices against abortion. So also the Lutheran forces that have permitted the same choice have been influenced by non-Lutheran liberal politics and ecumenical Christian views. These place higher premiums on freedom and self-determination. Neither line is a chemically pure retention of a thought-out Lutheran tradition in this matter any more than the various sides in respect to other health and medicine issues. A tradition is exposed to its environment and imparts something to it while taking something from it.

It must be said that the antiabortion forces in Lutheranism are far more organized than the prochoice movement and agencies. They have taken the initiative. Someone who would remain as objective as possible in recounting the issue is likely to agree with me in saying that they have amassed arguments and have articulated them well—though sometimes with passion and emotionalism that defeat their purpose. They have often shifted the burden of proof to those who draw on other aspects of the Lutheran tradition to allow for numerous circumstances in which there could be abortions.

By no means are all liberal Lutherans "proabortion." Most people, however, who allow for abortion have connected their thought with liberal political arguments. Liberalism has allowed itself to be preoccupied with the issue of choice so much that it has undervalued the importance of reflection on the issue of life. Until it does so, it will find itself avoiding many elements in the Lutheran understanding and will remain on the defensive. Choice, says the tradition, is not the only issue.

Several Lutheran bodies in America have felt called to charter formal studies and sometimes to make statements on the issue. Perhaps the most ambitious is a series of statements approved by the American Lutheran Church in 1974, 1976, and 1980. The 1974 statement stresses that the church body's position "is a pro-life position." It admits that there are very few Scriptural passages which bear directly on abortion. Referring to often-cited passages like Psalm 139:13–16, Job 10:9–11, Isaiah 44:2 and Jeremiah 1:5 the drafters say that these "help to inform the discussion, but have not led to consensus on the specific issues." Such dismissals have angered some of the more militant "pro-life" church members who *have* employed such passages explicitly.

The American Lutheran Church statements argue that "our confessional position as Lutherans requires that we ground any doctrinal statements on the Word of God as presented in our symbolical books," the ancient and Lutheran creeds, but notes that none of these contain any reference to abortion. Yet Lutheran views on God as creator, on living with laws in society, on having to act in a world of sin where choices are not always happy and forgiveness is necessary, and on the emphasis that human life demands respect at all levels, have something to say on the abortion issue.

The American Lutheran statements are tightly reasoned, judicious, full of concern for counselors, people facing difficult choice, and victims of injustice or the poor. The "pro-life" stand is clear but not dogmatically absolutist. It is that fact which has led the drafters of the statements and the leaders of the denomination to come under fire from those who very forcefully oppose abortion on what they insist are biblical grounds.[4]

Among Lutheran groups that have taken forthright antiabortion positions is the Missouri Synod. This body generally rejects political engagement. Here it has begun to intervene on the political issue and set out to equip its members to fight against abortion. Its denominational statements have been articulate and forceful.

In the Lutheran tradition, its commission statement begins with theology and puts medical and legal questions second. All three sections of the document "are agreed on the point that nontherapeutic abortion is wrong," though there are differences in nuance. Another characteristic element in its Lutheran approach is the fact that it says "men who are motivated by love of God and faith in Jesus Christ do not need a detailed set of rules to follow slavishly." Nor, it goes on, do they expect the biblical revelation to provide a specific regulation on every conceivable facet of an ethical problem. They seek general principles.

The statement acknowledges that abortion is not a simple issue. It requires evaluation and judgment. Life is a gift from God. The authors cite three verses from scripture that, they say, show that "life in the womb must be thought of in terms of personal being" (Exod. 21:22-24, Jer. 1:5, Luke 1:41). These are traditional texts for the point in Lutheranism. Second, "nascent life is of special value before God," and it is also designed to inherit eternal life. This section does acknowledge that nascent life that is a threat to the mother *may* have to be taken. Third, "fulfillment" is a goal of human life, and other humans should not interrupt the trajectory toward fulfillment. "Not wanting to be a mother does not provide a proper justification for deciding to have an abortion." Fulfillment demands a kind of trust in God, which abortion thwarts. The statement recognizes ambiguity and the demand for counsel and choice in cases of incest and rape. Never is there to be any allowance simply because of "even very grave psychiatric considerations." Fourth, life and death belong to the province of God.

With a finesse that many antiabortion arguments lack, the statement makes a distinction on the issue of "murder":

> The commandment "Thou shall not kill" was given specifically to forbid murder, that is, killing with hatred or malice or forethought. It is hardly proper, therefore, to make a direct application of this commandment to every act of abortion, since no hatred or malice may be involved in a given case. Nevertheless, it must be kept in mind that life comes into being as a special creative act of God, and no gift of His can be either rejected or destroyed with impunity. Any decision on the issue of abortion must take this last point with utmost seriousness.

Then, with a Lutheran regard for aftermaths, the statement acknowledges that there can be mistakes in judgment and thus "full assurance of forgiveness." However, it urges that availability of divine pardon suffers flagrant abuse whenever it is taken for granted.

As far as the legal side is concerned, the Missouri commission devoted itself more to complaining about the relaxing of older legal strictures than about imposing new ones, although latterly the synod has spoken also in favor of new restrictions. The medical section of the document calls on Christian physicians to be most scrupulous of all in this matter. The need for therapeutic abortions, it argues, is very rare. Seldom are there confirmable reasons for suspicion that an abnormal child will come forth.

As is often the case with such statements, because of the sparseness of past explicit Lutheran comment on an issue whose contemporary details no one could anticipate, this one nowhere explicitly evokes Luther, the Lutheran Confessions, or the traditions. But it acts Lutheranly in its modes of argument and its stresses. By no means is it a last word from the generally antiabortion part of the tradition, but it was one of the more effective first words. To say more at this point would be to distort the proportions and intentions of this book, which devotes itself to the whole of life, not to the fate of previable fetal life, however urgent that question is.[5]

THE ROLE OF BAPTISM

The rite of passage associated with the birth of a child for Lutherans is holy baptism. Almost without question Lutherans have practiced infant baptism to mark this first transit, this first passage across a *limen* or threshold. Some have made therapeutic connections with baptism. A hint of this is present in Ralph E. Peterson's 1982 commissioned statement for the Lutheran Church in America:

> The sacraments are essential to the healing ministry. Baptism gives us a new birth in Christ, the genuine life of God. This new life is made possible by "the seal of the gift of the Holy Spirit." This chrismation, in which the candidate's body is anointed with oil, has been restored in our most recent American Lutheran liturgy. "It is God also who has set his seal upon us as a pledge of what is to come and has given the Spirit to dwell in our hearts" (II Corinthians 1:22).

The chrismation with oil, it must be said, has been rare. It is hardly representative of the larger Lutheran tradition. Though it has some possibilities, it is not likely soon to become a central focus.[6]

Students of the theology and anthropology of baptism, who view it against history and similar rites in other faiths, have seen it as lustration or washing and cleansing. It is an agency for passage—Israel passed through the Red Sea, Jesus came up from the Jordan, Noah was saved on the ark. Lutheran liturgies often incorporate these motifs. Still, no Lutheran has claimed medicinal value for the water of baptism. Its washing was not intended to be of hygienic character any more than rising from baptism was anything more than analogous to literal lifesaving from drowning. If anything, the Lutheran tradition has underplayed the natural contexts of baptism, hurrying as it did to stress both the instrumental and pictorial parts it played in forgiveness and the new life. In other words, for Lutherans baptism *does* something. In faith it works forgiveness of sins. And it *shows* something. The Christian emerges from water as Christ emerged from the grave, to newness.

Luther's *Large Catechism* does use a therapeutic comparison or analogy, one that opens the door to seeing baptism as part of the search for being well in the wholistic sense.

> ... the blessings of Baptism are so boundless that if timid nature considers them, it may well doubt whether they could all be true. Suppose there was a physician who had such skill that people would not die, or even though they died would afterward live forever. Just think how the world would snow and rain money upon him. Because of the pressing crowd of rich men no one else could get near him. Now, here in Baptism there is brought free to every man's door just such a priceless medicine which swallows up death and saves the lives of all men.

So Christians are to draw "strength and comfort from it" when their sins or conscience oppress them. And there is a somatic tie:

> Since the water and the Word together constitute one Baptism, body and soul shall be saved and live forever: the soul through the Word in which it believes, the body because it is united with the soul and apprehends Baptism in the only way it can. No greater jewel, therefore, can adorn our body and soul than Baptism....

Martin Luther in the same catechism elaborates on what baptism does and signifies:

> This act or observance consists in being dipped into the water, which covers us completely, and being drawn out again. These two parts, being dipped under the water and emerging from it, indicate the power and effect of Baptism, which is simply the slaying of the old Adam and the resurrection of the new man, both of which actions must continue in us our whole life long. Thus a Christian life is nothing else than a daily Baptism, once begun and ever continued.

So the external sign has been appointed not only on account of what it confers, but also on account of what it signifies.

Lutheran theology of baptism thus provides the basis for vocation and calling. It urges freedom from the past, readiness to see guilt purged, and openness to the New Creation. The tradition now awaits a further extension of its theology of baptism into therapeutic understandings, given the impetus in the original documents for relating the act to both soul and body.[7]

THE STAGES OF DEVELOPMENT

In the next passage of life, from infancy to childhood, Lutheranism and its tradition have taken more interest in pedagogy or teaching than in developing specifically therapeutic understandings. Of course, its accent on trust underscores the ground for childhood development. Baptism connects with personality. The child is to be helped in garnering and defining an identity, without which well-being is impossible. The pedagogy includes accents on care of the body as a temple of the spirit, but there is not much distinctive about the Lutheran way of doing this. Are there distinctives in the roots of the tradition?

In *Luther's House of Learning: Indoctrination of the Young in the German Reformation* Gerald Strauss one-sidedly explores the ambiguities, intentions, and failures of Luther and his colleagues in respect to children. The reformers had only adult perceptions of childhood, uninformed by modern research into the stages of life. Yet, as Strauss points out, Luther and his peers were prescient in showing some interest in these topics. The closeness of disease and death to the world of children conditioned many of the adult attitudes. Thus, records of school rooms in the period give testimony to tragedy as in the case of the Strassburg school board in 1541: "Magister Sebastian lost 36 children and has only 28 left now. Magister Hartman: about 40 of his children have died; he has 43 left, but because of the dying has closed his school."

Strauss credits Luther for his open and warmhearted empathy for children, whose world he could and did enter. At the same time he and his co-workers made much of the absence of innocence in children and of their need for grace. In 1533 Andreas Osiander had to worry about letting emotions prevent the adult world from disciplining children. Theologians found it important to paint grim pictures of children's inclinations to evil and their achievement of evil acts. They set up a drastic picture and called for drastic means to bring a child to fulfillment. The writings include "a rasping tone and bilious vituperation" uncalled-for by circumstances. Yet there was always ambivalence. Luther himself showed it: "Children live in innocence.... They know no sin, they live without greed,... they will take an apple as cheerfully as a coin."

Along with many authors of his day, Luther believed that stages of life come in sevens. At seven, the child is moving from innocence toward manifest guilt. At age fourteen, Luther observed the physical and psychological assaults that came with awakening to sexuality. No apparent innocence is left. The Reformers wanted to delay the acceptance of sexual maturity, to postpone acknowledgment of sexuality. Hence, there were boarding schools, if only for the elite few, which were sex-segregated.

Yet Luther also recognized the psychological harm done by sexual repression. Sex "is a necessary and natural thing. Every man needs a woman, every woman must have a man." Satisfying sexual wants is "more urgent than eating, drinking,... sleeping and waking." Again, "Nature will out. It wants to spurt its seed." The pedagogical literature of the early Lutheran decades busied itself with plots to keep sexual stimulants—dancing, plays, sensual excitements, mingling of sexes, and the like—from children. The children made their own contribution to the Lutheran tradition by compensating and evidently thinking *more* about sex. So, at least, suggests the literature! And their leaders counseled hard work to help the young forget their sexual drives.[8]

Thus, the preoccupation in respect to infancy and childhood was discipline and in respect to adolescence was sexuality. Whatever else the Lutheran tradition began to say or do to diagnose the mental, spiritual, or physical problems of people in these passages, they concentrated their attention on these major themes. In this book, which is not about "passages" but about the overall tradition, we cannot trace in detail what was said about each passage. The purpose here is simply to see how Lutheran understandings of what a human being was in the light of God's purpose colored all the therapeutic counsel.

As for the middle life—did one speak of a mid-life crisis, or was any part of mid-life *not* a crisis to the Reformers?—almost all the literature is addressed to this age group. Marriage, expressions of sexuality, care of health, parental responsibilities were elements for the middle of life. They were the main subjects of Lutheran counsel, as all the rest of the book makes clear. The themes related to aging are comprehended in subjects which we shall deal with in a chapter on death and dying.

HOLY COMMUNION AT ALL LATER STAGES

One combined theme deserves treatment. Having connected the care of the young to the sacrament of baptism, it remains to connect the care of the adolescent and the adult to the other sacrament, Holy Communion. Until recent reforms in modern Lutheranism, this was also connected with the rite of confirmation. As Frank W. Klos pointed out in *Confirmation and First Communion*, Martin Luther made little of what later became a kind of adolescent rite in the eyes of many. He rejected it as a sacrament and made much of making little of it as a rite. Nor did he practice it. He found no New Testament command or promise connected with the practice, and he feared that it might detract from the daily recall of baptism. The tradition, however, lived on. Since Luther did not discourage the practice, "for three centuries, Luther's followers experimented," seeking to find a proper rite and understanding. A modern commission classified the experiments in six categories, none of them directly related to our theme of well-being.

What *is* interesting is that so much experiment was necessary because Lutherans felt a need, which anthropologists have confirmed, for some sort of adolescent rite of passage. This hunch is confirmed in modern times when one reads the rationales of American Lutherans for confirmation when youths are in the tenth grade. As Klos elaborates, most of it is related to psychologically informed studies of stages and passages. He quotes Michael Argyle: adolescence is "a time of religious choice." There is discussion of the "freedom to become," of "patterns of growth," particularly on the subject of becoming sexually mature. The commission cited Erik Erikson on adolescence as a time of personality integration. As Jean Piaget also showed the Lutherans, mental operations change. Without using the term *rites de passage*, the official panel clearly showed the influence of such a designation. Wherever confirmation belongs theologically, there must always be some passage over a threshold, a separation, a merging, a reintegration. The therapeutic implications are fairly obvious.[9]

Whether communion connects with confirmation or not, it becomes the sacrament for the adult and aged stages of life. Although one returns daily to baptism for a new beginning, in the Lord's Supper one regularly returns for strength. Ralph Peterson is a bit ambiguous about what he means, but he clearly wants to evoke bodily understandings when he says:

> The sacraments are essential to the healing ministry.... The new life in Christ and the Holy Spirit in the Church is nourished and sustained in the mystery of the Eucharist, the Holy Communion.... For the Christian there is no life *or health* without it. (Emphasis mine.)

He concludes:

> So it is that in the great Lutheran tradition of the ministry of pastoral counseling and soul care, illness and suffering have been seen in the context of the mystery of victorious life in the Body of Christ.

Peterson's ambiguity is not out of place. It has roots in the beginnings of the tradition. No one will understand the Lutheran concept of the Lord's Supper or of healing unless he or she recognizes the way the concept of health turns from the spiritual into the wholistic. The spiritual is always primarily meant, but Lutheranism does not picture well-being if there is not spiritual health. One cannot do more for the whole person than to help nurture the health of the person before God. The code name for this tie was "the soul."[10]

This tradition does not constantly stress the ancient church's frequent references to the Lord's Supper as a medicine for immortality. Nor does it stress the physical result of nourishment with the transformed molecules of bread. The concept was in every case more spiritual or, Lutherans would say, "sacramental." Thus in the *Large Catechism*, "it is appropriately called the food of the soul since it nourishes and strengthens the new man." Through baptism "our human flesh and blood have not lost their old skin." We "grow weary and faint," but "the Lord's Supper is given as a daily food and sustenance. . . . For the new life should be one that continually develops and progresses." Several pages later Luther again writes in a document that has become official for the church:

> We must . . . regard the sacrament . . . as a pure, wholesome, soothing medicine which aids and quickens us *in both soul and body. For where the soul is healed, the body has benefited also.* Why, then, do we act as if the sacrament were a poison which would kill us if we ate of it? (Emphasis mine.)[11]

With its horror of magical concepts of anything physical, such as the elements of bread and wine in the Lord's Supper, later Lutheranism has never fully developed this clear and basic insight of the *Large Catechism*. The Lutheran manuals of pastoral care have often been uninformed by sacramental thinking. Most sacramental writing in Lutheranism has shown concern for doctrine and worship more than for use and effect. In the process it has often ended up with a somewhat cold, breadless, bloodless approach that offers less than what Martin Luther and the early confessors saw in the meal. In the underlined words of the *Large Catechism* on the Lord's Supper one can find the beginning of a whole charter for Lutheran psychosomatic concerns. This may be the most underdeveloped aspect of the tradition. Almost nothing could be closer to its center.

·9·

The Completion of Being, the Meaning of Dying

The faith traditions do not have something clear to say on many topics devoted to health and medicine, but there is at least one great exception. Most of them have devoted much attention to the theme of death and dying. They may not all be expert on or occupied with distinctive approaches to human care or the passages of life. Yet whoever ventures to speak or act in the field of religion has to have thought through what the end of life means for the living of life. Not that the traditions within Christianity are at all points different from each other. Ours is not a pursuit of uniquenesses but of distinctives. Through the centuries the traditions pick up much from their cultures. They tend to fuse and become confused. Even at the point of their origins they draw on common roots—be these biblical, Catholic, or whatever. Yet the early words of a tradition stamp something of what is said later. In a vital heritage, what is said about death will link up with the heart of faith.

Most literature on well-being deals with the living of life apart from death. Death is the termination of life, of being. Yet in religious traditions it is not simply termination of life as known, but it can mean the transforming of life, or as I prefer to speak of it—out of the many choices that the modern literature offers—as "the completion of being." Faith traditions have found it necessary persistently to take the question of death from the margins of life or from the recesses of the mind and bring it to the forefront. All of life on the religious horizon is a "being toward death." To evade this is to eliminate the possibility of true well-being through the years of life.

The Bible, from almost the first to the very last pages, has an extremely frank and realistic approach to death. The subject is a constant. On Christian soil through most of the centuries there was an engrossment with the topic—sometimes almost to the point of the morbidly fascinating and even the grotesque. Students of the subject of death, most notably Philip Aries in *The Hour of Our Death*,[1] have found in the arts, the folklore, and the behavioral patterns of Christians an astounding variety of attitudes and practices. Clearly, there is no way to write a simple book on "death in the Christian tradition." The Lutheran tradition has also known many variations in the different periods and places in which it has found expression. Our interest has to do only with what connects with the concept of well-being.

Most modern writers on the subject bewail the fact that contemporaries have made death a taboo subject, one from which to escape. In reaction against nineteenth-century morbidity, people in the twentieth century have set out to insulate themselves from the experience and thought of death. Violence on television or in the cinema may bring death close to home, but there is in it all a certain artificiality and distance. In other respects, death is pushed away. Grandparents do not live in the house with children, so the young do not see deterioration or aging to the point of death. Those with terminal illness are screened from view in clinics and hospitals. A few minutes after an automobile accident, everything is re moved from sight, including bodies and blood from the highway. The cosmetic industry promotes the illusion of perpetual youth. Even as the culture comes to put more of a premium on aging, this occurs apart from the theme of death.

Thanks to the persistence and eloquence of some researchers and writers, however, this situation has begun to change to some extent. Elisabeth Kübler-Ross and Ernest Becker, for two examples, have warred against what Becker calls "the denial of death," in the book of the same name.[2] Kübler-Ross taught a generation to observe a sequence of stages in the processes of dying.[3] Philip Aries has awakened interest in the history of cultural attitudes and artifacts. The day may soon come when death is a voguish topic. There is much talk of a "meaningful death," "death with dignity," and "a happy death." To put a name on something feared is to begin to tame it, to domesticate it. These therapeutic efforts at naming have generally been welcomed in the churches, including within the Lutheran tradition.

WHAT LUTHERAN FAITH HAS TO SAY

At the same time, such research, since it occurs in secular academic or clinical settings, does not address itself directly to what faiths have to say in particular. Seminarians, pastors, lay leaders, and therapists are more likely to acquire their views of death and dealing with it from people who have no knowledge of their traditions than from their progenitors. Thomas Aquinas, Martin Luther, John Calvin, or even modern Christian writers on death such as Ladislaus Boros, S.J., or John Hick, are not consulted in most therapies. Yet to minister to people on subjects of well-being without seeing how their faith connects with death as the completion of being is to avoid major resources. It is to lead toward contradictions or to promote escapism.

Certain common elements in Christian treatments of death impinge upon Lutheran understandings. With all of Christendom, there is in Lutheran settings a serious attempt to do justice to the biblical writings. This means, for example, that there is a dealing with the Old Testament's realism about death and its horizon without much reference to a life to come. Second, with all Christianity, Lutheranism asserts that death does not have the last word or the final victory. It is not an ultimate sting. What God has done in Jesus Christ is to numb the power of death without removing death, to assure that the God of love continues to enwrap the believer beyond the confines of mortal existence. The last line of the creed, "I believe in the resurrection of the body," seems to flow inevitably from the first, "I believe in God the Father Almighty."

Lutheranism shared the general Christian creedal affirmation of this resurrection of the body, whatever it has come to mean in different times. Certainly the modern scientific understandings of atoms, molecules, chemical processes, and the like have colored images of what the new life with God after death could mean. New physical understandings have replaced Ptolemaic and Copernican images of the geography and furniture of a heaven or a hell as places of fulfillment or suffering after death. Yet there has been no wavering on the central "yes" to life that goes with the belief in resurrection.

Of course, most Americans believe in some form of being after physical death. Usually this is phrased as "immortality," though that is not the best way to put biblical, Christian, or Lutheran understandings. In opinion polls, the general population "generally" believes in immortality, whereas the Lutheran percentage is much higher. Yet in the general culture this belief is quite vague, unclothed with enough reality for it to inform the search for well-being.

Lutherans have generally shown little interest in laboratory research about life after death or philosophical discussions of immortality. They make resurrection and what it stands for an article of faith and find reports from "the other side" unconvincing and sterile. A book of purported "messages from beyond" from a well-known Lutheran theologian through a medium to his daughter raised almost no churchly curiosity at all. It was not regarded as a sign of hope or a testimony to Christian belief, but as a cultural curiosity.

The vagueness in religious circles and the general culture has meant that as Lutheran leadership trains itself to understand death and dying, the whole concept of "the completion of being" and the fulfillment of life in the resurrection moves to the margins. This, therefore, means that much of the clinical literature and pastoral training discusses the Lutheran tradition without reference to what follows death. Of course, this is a serious distortion, since the tradition has been so consistent in promoting well-being by reference to the fact that by the grace of God in Christ, death does not have the last word.

This is anomalous because in the daily ministry of congregations and pastors to the dying, and then to the grieving circle, hope for the resurrection is central. Countless aged Christians in nursing homes long for death "to be with" their departed spouse or other loved ones. At graveside the grand New Testament words about reunion and new life ring clearly. In the course of counsel to the bereaved, the recognition of continued life in the resurrection appears regularly. People who have to come to terms with the presence of death hear words of assurance about the continuity of love in the life lived under God. Yet observers regularly note that these affirmations have a double effect. One set of Christians permits the belief to grow so vague that it does little to remove the sting of death. The other set, perhaps a minority today, uses the promise to evade death and realism about contemporary living.

The salutary aspect of this vagueness about belief in what follows death lies in the fact that, among people who are not escapists, the brutal reality of death remains especially strong. When people are forced to face up to it, they stand the best chance of coming to well-being through the years *before* death. The Lutheran tradition is consistent in its counsel that death is to be regarded, remembered, reckoned with, not only at the point of dying but daily through life. That theme comes close to being at the center of the Lutheran tradition on death, yet it is generally expressed without much morbidity.

WHEN CARE COMES INTO PLAY

The Lutheran approach is not highly distinctive, as far as practice is concerned. Take an instance of a believer who has a terminal illness. She becomes the subject of ministry by the congregation just as she is to find a new vocation in suffering and prayer. Intercessory prayer is at the heart of the mutual ministry. This becomes palpable until "the communion of saints" is felt.

Where pastoral ministry is effective, the ministers will make regular calls on the person who is ill. They will help her come to terms with her destiny, yet without constant recourse to the theme of physical death. They bring greetings from the congregation, assurances of support, and inquiry about physical or other needs. Along with the more technical sides of counsel, there will almost always be a form of communication that relies on the Word of God and issues in joint prayer. Frequently, the minister will extend the Lord's Table into the sickroom. There will be celebration of Holy Communion, with its explicit references to Jesus' dying and victory.

Meanwhile, if the congregation is living out its Lutheran vocation, it moves into action. The well-supported member will have friends who represent the gathering and do not come only as individuals to visit. They may receive some informal counsel as to how to help the person cope with the impending death—and are likely to report back as to how they themselves have been ministered *to*. Many a congregation has been strengthened by the witness that nothing separated the person, not even death, from the love of God in Christ. Love is stronger than death, faith is weightier than doubt, and hope transcends present circumstances. Many a parish will have a deacon or some other "other-than-natural friend" call. This is considered important because it suggests that the whole congregation, including those who are not related to or close friends of the dying person, are involved. Some parishes have trained callers, not to impersonalize or render technical the act of support, but to be of help to the dying one.

In Lutheran as in other Christian congregations there occur daily acts of concern that can never be chronicled, so common that they do not make news. Does the ill person need chauffeurs to bring relatives to the hospital? Baby-sitters at home? Legal help? Is there a place for flowers, a smuggled bottle of wine "for the stomach's sake," for books? There may be a flood of greeting cards. The Sunday church bulletin with its prayer list is an almost constant transmitter of news between patient and congregation.

All of this may look ordinary, almost trivial, only humane, a mere Christianization of what thoughtful people do in their clubs or ethnic groups. The Lutheran congregation does not take that suggestion as a judgment on itself, but feels judged when it fails to do as well as those in the surrounding world. It may also descend into sentimentality or the creation of an unwelcome "busyness." Some people as they move toward death would just as soon be given some quiet and time to do some of their own coping. Yet instinct, manners, taste, and technical know-how can combine to make congregational support a positive element in the search for well-being.

The larger point is that all of this is *not* trivial, but is the stuff of life itself. It relates to a central Lutheran theme, stated in the kind of paradoxical or contradictory form that Lutherans cherish. The believer dies very much alone, *and* the believer dies in company. On the aloneness, we shall have more to say in a moment. In regard to the company, there are two affirmations. First, while Jesus Christ with his "My God, My God, why hast thou forsaken me?" experienced and expressed abandonment by God, he alone was abandoned. God's raising of Jesus assured that never again would one identified with Jesus in faith be abandoned. All would suffer, death would come, but dying would be in company, the company of Christ.

The other company is human, contemporary. Through the extended Eucharist or Lord's Supper in congregation and sickroom, through intercessory prayer, through pastoral and lay visitations, the dying person becomes aware that her struggle is shared, she is supported, and she is ministered to by those not momentarily in her circumstance. Here as so often we have to insist that for Lutherans there is not too much that can be said about the tradition's contribution to well-being in the case of people who do not undertake the discipline of what Dietrich Bonhoeffer, in his book of the same name, called "life together." In his terms stated elsewhere, Christ exists "as community," in the congregation, and is present in the life of the *Gemeinde*, the gathering.[4] One does not join a congregation at the time of the announcement of a terminal illness—though he or she is always welcome to, and will then also be ministered to. Instead, if there is concern for well-being, one undertakes the common life with other Christians in the midst of apparent health and sees it then enriched, ripened, and naturally expressed in times of crisis.

Alone. Luther wrote, "We have all been ordered to die, and no one will be able to die for another. But each one will be obliged to contend against death in his own person." Are we *only* alone? "We may be able to shout into one another's ears, but each one will have to be fit for himself at the time of death. I shall not be with you, nor you with me." For that reason, Christians had to equip themselves. They learned to "shout in the ears" and thus pray with the dying person. Believers do not, dare not, desert the dying. At least a representative of the human race, the Christian Church, the circle of family and friends, or the congregation is there as a "shouter." "No Christian," added Luther, "should doubt at his end that he is not alone when dying, but he should be confident that very many eyes are looking at him." These are the eyes of God, Christ, angels, saints, and the congregation. "A Christian should envisage this and should have no doubt regarding it. This emboldens him to die."

Luther returns repeatedly to the tension between aloneness and dying in company. Heinrich Bornkamm relates the tradition to modern times in passages on this theme.[5] Christians have a good reputation about knowing how to die, but they have a bad reputation for knowing how to live. They are experts on the eternal and have lost their eye on the temporal. Thus Luther says we "view this temporal life only through a painted glass, blinkingly, as it were; but we view yonder eternal life with clear, open eyes." That is why from the beginning Lutheran articulators have stressed the realism of aloneness in death and the need for company.

WHEN DEATH COMES

Death comes. Lutheran disposal of the body and ministering to the bereaved soon look generally Christian, though sometimes overwhelmed by current cultural practices. Not all of these are necessarily congruent with the Lutheran tradition. They may blur and blunt its clear effects. There may be cremation, now that people no longer see it as a challenge by agnostics to a God who could only with difficulty "reconstruct" or "resuscitate." Cremation is coming to be seen as a good expression of biblical realism—"ashes to ashes, dust to dust." In more and more families it is seen as a witness to the Bible, to nature, to contemporaries—and a mark of the "stewardship of the earth." It remains a minority expression in Lutheranism, however, so we do well to focus on the ordinary attempts to promote well-being through funerary rites.

Among the host of morticians there is an appropriate number of Lutherans. Many of them are sensitive to the demands of faith among the survivors. Yet they are not always imaginative, free from cultural bonds, or economically motivated to help families give expression to the core faith as held in their tradition. Almost every time embalming occurs, the cosmetic effect becomes important, and the setting of the funeral home works against confronting death and the heart of the Christian hope. The illusion of continuing life is sought. Soft lights, constant Muzak, hushed conversations at a "wake"—all may have therapeutic value. They may also appear in discontinuity with what is said at funeral rites and at graveside.

Historically, Lutheran burial has been from the church. The retraditioning movement is encouraging that last rites be held there. The sanctuary provides for the eucharistic setting, and this can be seen as a great celebrative act of "saints above and saints below." The mortuary is far less congenial for this purpose. Burial from the church can allow for all the evocative symbols of the life that goes on day by day, week by week—instead of the artificial and disruptive or discontinuous symbolization one finds in the funeral chapel. Often the church setting allows for members of the congregation to provide what we might call "the sacrament of the coffee

cup" for people as they return from the burial site. It discourages grandilo-
quent eulogy; the person who has died has been part of these people, this
place. There is no compulsion to have to certify this nervously, verbally.

Graveside rites, usually read out of a Lutheran book of worship, share
much with the church ecumenical. They depart from the tradition if anything that there occurs blunts the reality of death or minimizes the hope of
resurrection. Those are the two constants in Lutheran ministry to the
grieving. Then begins the continuation of ministry. "Teach us to number
our days" is the graveside legacy. The brighter sides involve the reincor-
poration of the survivors into the life of the community, the occasioning of
moments of cheer. There will be offers of physical aid, perhaps of economic support, the proffering of services. Most of all, one cheers at the notion that those who have gone through the experience serve the memory of
the dead best by living, by being of service to those who have served them.
Life goes on as the members look ahead to the only certain fact about their
mortal existence: they *will* die.

DEATH AS A CHALLENGE TO MEANING

Those homey and homely depictions of folk and congregational life deal
chiefly with behavior patterns, which may or may not hook in integrally to
the substance of a faith tradition. Yet for the long hours during which one
person faces death and the longer hours during which others are "number-
ing their days" and living their lives, it is the substance of the tradition that
matters. Death is the great challenge to meaning. It is arbitrary, cruel,
never truly welcome. How, in its face, can one witness to the steadfast love
of a God who has power to give and control and extend life? Are we in a
random universe? Is death an illusion? Is it not merely the completion of
being but the threat to *all* meaning? While we see funeral practices connected with those of the culture as a whole, we look for distinctives when
we see how a tradition interprets life and offers understandings of death.
Here Lutheranism has much to say.

One of its sayings focuses on a contradiction already mentioned: one dies
in company, yes, but one also dies alone. Here the tradition begins with
Luther, who never tired of reminding himself and others of this aspect of
"being toward death." It is obvious that death is alone, that it is personal,
and yet the obvious is often forgotten, especially in church, theology, and
therapy. When death is generalized and people are taught just to see it as
part of the universal natural experience—which it also is—they are de-
prived of aspects of its meaning.

A popular modern Lutheran thinker, on whom we shall rely for some distinctives, Helmut Thielicke, stresses the point. First he quotes a stinging reminder from another near-contemporary thinker, Alfred E. Hoche, who wrote in 1936:

> It is a curious drama that man, who knows the supreme and inescapable law about the cessation of every life all around him and of every life that has ever been lived, still finds it personally oppressive to yield to that law. The notion strikes him as unbearable that this fantastic subjective world that he carries within himself, and that exists in this particular shape but once in time, should simply be wiped out. It is unbearable simply to collapse at the side of the road while the others travel on, conversing as though nothing had happened. . . . The vividness of this feeling . . . makes mockery of all logic.

That states the issue; Luther, at the beginning, thundered the point home as the first word.

In the tradition, death is not merely the result of natural law. It is a crisis, a decisive event. I am partly responsible for it. I have taken actions against God—even if I have seemed to be "saintly"—and am thus an agent of what is ahead of me. Somehow what is happening is also my due. This is a particularly uncomfortable aspect of the Lutheran view of death, but without it the therapy and affirmation this version of faith offers is hollow. One must first have its problem in order to make sense of its partial solutions. God addresses me, the "Thou" speaks to this "I" even, and especially, in this dire act. Some sermons may have been aimed at the world, the congregation; this message has my name on it, and I am being tested to see if I can read and apply it. Death is a limit and a boundary, a reminder that I am not God who sets limits and boundaries. It is also a sign of my rebellion. I wanted to cross the limits and boundaries to create a Godward horizon on my own. That was futile.

Another Lutheran, Carl Stange, put this well:

> We see that God speaks for us in our conscience from the fact that death carries out the verdict already spoken in our conscience—and we see that death comes from God in the fact that because of our sin we stand in fear of death.

When I hear Paul say that "the wages of sin is death," it shocks. So Luther:

> This verse reveals in striking fashion that death in man is in countless ways a far greater calamity than the death of other living beings. . . . The death of human beings is a genuine disaster. . . . The reason is that man is being created for this purpose: to live forever in obedience to the Word and to be like God. He was not created for death.

Therefore, it shocks him to know that something has gone wrong, and he is now destined for death.

Death, therefore, does not sting so much as a mere physical event, a part of natural biology, but as an aspect of the relation between God and the human. It is, says Lutheranism, not so much an issue of nature or processes, but of history and events. I do not die as an animal but as one who has to come to terms with being only man when I wanted to be God. I am dust and to dust I shall return. We join the animals in the march to dust, but we are really different, for the God who marked our limits and boundaries addresses us personally, distinctly. "Adam, where art thou?" Luther liked to speak of the human being "alone, alone, all alone" in the death situation. It is unmistakable, when I die alone: God is addressing me, not someone else.

Helmut Thielicke lifts up for moderns the roots of the Lutheran tradition when he stresses the contrast between animal death and the shocking unnatural fact of human dying. Luther speaks of *mors in homine*, death in man, not the death *of* man. Death *in* us, as part of our being, is a more shattering disaster than the death *of* the animals. They die oblivious to the character of God, unpuzzled over their "mistreatment," unaware of the reasons for their treatment. They are not aware of a God who has reason to set boundaries, to be angry with what humans do with those boundaries. Yes, Luther says, a hog at the point of slaughter expresses distress, but this is only physically induced pain. Human death is worse, because it has to be aware of the meaning of the pain.

When I die, I am threatened not only because I give up mortal life, but I also surrender my company with God. Were that not the case, Luther says, death would "truly be a kind of sleep." But it is more and other than sleep. "If we were compelled," says Luther, "to look forward only to [physical] death, we might say with the poet [Martial]: 'Neither fear, nor long for, the last day.' So I cannot by myself cope with what is happening to me."

The substance of this personal view has its counterpart in the personal character of the victory over death. Thielicke quotes Luther on Christ, who died and transcended boundaries and limits through the activity of God. This Christ is my exemplar, the first to go through what I now do. "Mine are Christ's living, doing, and speaking, his suffering and dying, mine as much as if I had lived, done, spoken, suffered, and died as he did." Through baptism, of which the Lutheran tradition never tires of speaking as it addresses death and resurrection, I am linked with what happens to Christ. Hence, also, victory, completion of being, becomes completion of well-being.

In this understanding, eternal life has already begun, to the degree that

I live "in Christ." Now biological death is not seen simply as the result of the wrath of a just God, for that wrath has been turned aside in Christ, through faith in God's grace. Personal death has lost its sting. Some measure of anxiety can now disappear. To the congregation of the faithful, it has lost this dimension of its meaningfulness. The one who is to die dies with Christ and somehow experiences Christ's rising. Here the personal hope tied to the awareness of death as a personal event heals just as the facing of death shocked: I am not part of undifferentiated being, an element of immortal souldom. Whatever God has in store for me has my name on it. And things shall be well with me.

Another paradox in Lutheran understandings of death lives on through all its tradition into the present, in its education and worship life as well as in theology and practical counsel. That is: with Christ the Victor as my exemplar, and with the sting of my terrible death thus removed, I have reason to be free of morbidity. I need not dwell on death, my death. Yet at the same time, this tradition more than most calls me to be aware of death. I can get nothing out of the themes and messages of the grace of God until and unless I apply the understanding of death to my every act, my daily doings.

Thus, this same tradition that allows none of its heirs to be paralyzed by death insists that the whole search for well-being must keep them from evading it. More positively, they should face it constantly. The presence of cemeteries around us does not fulfill this mission. Pagans also look at them and still find ways to minimize death. Thus the Stoics: where I am, death is not. Where death is, I am not. So where and since the two are not together, why should I concern myself with the death that is not where I am? For the Lutheran Christian, however, where death is, I am—death is *in homine*, in the human. If it is in me, it must be faced as a germ, as the plague, or I can never have well-being. Luther addressing himself to ignorance, says, "This is the reason why everyone organizes his plans and projects as though he were going to live forever. Because of this common practice people transform their life into an eternal life." And yet, then, they *do* die.

Because "in the midst of life we are in death" and death is in us, death must, says Luther, be "ever present." For that reason the moment of death is not the only crisis, but instead the believer has to face up to the lifelong presence of "my death" now and constantly. Luther again says, ". . . fear of death is the death of the human soul. This fear, despair, horror is death itself." This is the theme taken up so eloquently by maverick Lutherans of the past two centuries, people such as Søren Kierkegaard and Paul Tillich. One could conceivably reduce and minimize the impact of the physical moment of death; it happens to many when they are unconscious and in sleep, or so suddenly they could not prepare. The problem is that death is constant, ever present.

In the Lutheran tradition there is very little interest in heroic death, in those who can thumb their noses at the presence of death. Luther thought that the human mind or reason was a factory that constantly generated ways to evade the divine boundaries. So in the present case, the philosophers counseled a reasonable contempt for death. "Since reason is determined to escape God's wrath, it proposes either the way of disdain [*contemptus*] or the way of blasphemy." Therefore of the Stoic, Luther can say, "What of it when Epicurus [who holds death in contempt] dies? He not only does not know that there is a God, but also fails to understand his own misery which he is experiencing." One might say, "Good for Epicurus; 'whatever gets you through the night....'" But for the Christian theologian there must be honesty, no contrivance; there must be awareness and knowledge.[6]

The address of victory is as personal as is death, and it all relies on the character of God and the exemplar, Jesus Christ. Luther stresses the promise. "Faith which relies on ... a promise and ventures joyously must be present. What sort of savior or god would he be who could not or would not save us from death, sin and hell? What the true God promises and carries out must be something big." The exemplar is decisive: "Just try to find yourself in Christ, and not in yourself; then you will find yourself eternally in Him." Whenever the Lutheran tradition has been true to itself while promoting wholeness, it has come to precisely this focus.

Well-being does not come when I expunge awareness of death or explain it away. It can come only when I refuse to put myself higher than God, when I accept the divine source of my death and its meaning. For reasons of which I am at least partly responsible, God has found reason to inflict death. Evading God means failing to find the divine victory, life replacing death *in homine*, in me. In this tradition, the search for well-being is a constant drama, full of events more than natural processes. I do not watch my hair and teeth fall out to understand the meaning of death. I observe the way I have not observed the limits and boundaries God has set. I note my transgressions. And I identify with Christ the exemplar. Still, with awareness of death being constant, life remains a historical process: "This life is not being whole, but becoming whole, not a rest, but an exercise.... It is not the end, but the way."[7]

Postscript

During the summer in which I was completing research on this book, the bishops of the Lutheran churches in America met for a week-long conference with their spouses at Keystone, Colorado. As a "theologian-in-residence" for the occasion, I also wore an interviewer's hat. On long bus rides, at table, or in their rooms, I interviewed the presidents of the larger Lutheran bodies concerning health and medicine in the Lutheran tradition.

James R. Crumley, Jr., is president of the Lutheran Church in America, David W. Preus is bishop of the American Lutheran Church, and William M. Kohn of the Association of Evangelical Lutheran Churches. A planned interview with Ralph Bohlmann, head of the Lutheran Church–Missouri Synod, never eventuated, but I have highlighted one of Bohlmann's emphases in discussing the First Article of the Creed in the *Large Catechism*. It is he who stresses that Luther sees "me" created "along with" all the rest of creation. I have tried to be sensitive to the Missouri Synod's separate tradition on these pages.

The three presidents were busy preparing for conventions in September at which their three bodies voted to form one new Lutheran church in America. During these years they have had special reasons to listen to their members, to poll congregants, to be in close touch with their pastors. At the same time, all three have deep roots in pastoral ministry and reputations for having overcome "bureaucratic remoteness" and having remained responsive to the life of their churches.

To interview them, then, is not to take an opinion poll of a Lutheran cross section. Yet it did allow for an attempt to see how three representative leaders saw their traditions in the context of present-day church life. I was able to incorporate their views into this draft, to use them to qualify my statements, or to be emboldened to make some generalizations that otherwise would have been stated more vaguely and meekly. It strikes me as valuable to close this book with direct reference to their views of the heart of the tradition, though the interviews brought up all the other chapter subjects of this book as well.

They all agreed with the root notions of Martin Luther about "wholistic" views. As the Lutheran epigraph to this book has it, "where the soul is healed, the body has benefited also." In their own words they vigorously reinforced the contention of Einar Billing. They believe that Luther and Lutheranism are best understood as "adhering to a common center and radiating out like the rays of the sun from one glowing core, the gospel of the forgiveness of sins." They also personalized their grasp of this core or central notion.

David Preus instantly connected "justification by faith" with the freedom and trust it brings to "well-being." "If it is in your gut," he said, "you are ready for everything." When ill health comes, you are more ready to "tough it out." Preus insisted that there was no "quick fix" in Lutheranism, no magic cure based on techniques of positive thinking. Physical well-being is *not* the highest value in life. Once one "gets that right," he or she is free for well-being.

Lutheranism, Preus went on, has its own way of promoting health through preventive care. Some of these modes include "singing songs, developing a blithe spirit." There is in this tradition a positive regard for the body; there is no room for docetism, for spiritualistic views that turn the faith into something ghostly, remote, uneasy with body.

Preus stressed the pastoral care dimensions of the tradition. Lutheranism is also not afraid to set norms and insist on them. Yet through confession and forgiveness it seeks to keep the standards and yet affirm the violator—which everyone is, daily. As for prayer, this faith does not develop special healing-prayer techniques and does not rely on miraculous cures, though it was Preus who kept insisting that the charismatics' approach was "within the allowable range" for Lutheranism. "For all Lutherans, there is no impulse to limit expectancy of miracle." Yet the normal intercessory prayer does not concentrate on supernatural interruptions so much as on the constancy of God, the support of the congregation, and the assurance that nothing shall separate us from the love of God.

With his colleagues, Preus stressed the role of the gathering, the congregation. In conversation with him we developed the formula that the best thing Lutheranism has to offer for the context of well-being in times of ill health is to have been a member of a warm congregation for some time! More positively, the counsel is to become a part of an intercessory prayer-minded fellowship that promotes and thrives on care. This is not to be done prudentially, for the sake of "rainy days" to come, but for intrinsic reasons. Yet support and care *will* occur in the bad times as part of the "things" that come to those who have sought first the Kingdom of God.

In the face of suffering, Preus again used the phrase "tough it out," but this toughing it out is done in serene confidence that beyond the pain, which one can never fully interpret, and in the midst of ambiguities and doubts, faith and trust will be upheld. And beyond all this is a Lutheran *ars moriendi*, a cultivated "art of dying." There is nothing world denying or morbid about the way the Lutheran is urged and taught to face death with both rage and equanimity, regret and confidence.

It is easy to see why, if their bishops are representative, the three bodies of Lutherans can come together, for the other two churchmen voiced in parallel terms many of the same interests and came to similar conclusions. The Preus conversation was the longest and most leisurely and my notes were most extensive. Yet notes from the other interviews turn up many accents that deserve separate treatment.

What is at the heart of the Lutheran expression of well-being? President Kohn: "Joy! the joy of living! the joy that comes with freedom, the freedom to give of one's self because so much has been given in the Gospel." For a fleeting moment conflicting images cross the mind: of gloomy-Dane Lutherans such as Søren Kierkegaard, of melancholy Swedes and Norwegians being pious about their Pietism, of dour Lutherans trudging sourly back from the eucharistic table, of lugubrious confessional hymns. Yet countering these are the images that do match Kohn's accent on "joy."

The Lutheran, he said, has not developed, on the other hand, a pasty-smiled personality type. The joy that goes with the forgiven life, the New Being in Christ, "speaks much to wellness." Again, the words were *confidence, trust, carefreeness, care.* Kohn admitted that the Lutheran tradition was at a disadvantage because it was hard to "sell." It offered no fads, no instant therapies, no supersitions, no charms. Yet he agreed with Preus that, hard as it is to get the church's easy message right, once one "got it right," all the rest could begin to follow. Here is not only a way of believing and thinking but also a way of life.

President Kohn made much of the Lutheran concept of dignity, of a self-esteem that is not achieved but derived, not earned but given—and, hence, more secure. We talked about the high view of humanity expressed in a Christmas hymn. There Christians praise God "who our race hath honored thus that He deigns to dwell with us." From this followed the equally high view of care: the Christian in this tradition is to be not *as* Christ but *a* Christ to the neighbor. Kohn was happy that Lutheranism has always encouraged medicine, has been open to scientific care and cure, has built hospitals and deaconess *Krankenhäuser*, but he did not want it to rest on old laurels. He hopes that it will continue to foster "mediating institutions" between the family and the large impersonal agencies of modern society.

With Preus, Kohn stressed the realism and frankness that Lutherans in-culcate in respect to suffering and death. There is in it a denial of the denial of death, yet this does not take the shape of morbid fascination with its power, since it has only the second last word.

Bishop Crumley, asked to comment on what struck him as the main cor-ollary of the central Lutheran theme, was as ready as were his two col-leagues. For him as for Luther the main accent in word and sacraments is the phrase "for you." The body and blood are given "for you." The Word is not Word until it moves from the merely intellectual or propositional to the lively connection with "you." One comes to this through a view of con-fidence in a God who cares for all, and for all of me—including my body. With this comes a confident view of the self. If I had talked to a president one hundred years ago would I have heard this accent? It has been latent in Lutheranism, but it may have taken modern theology and therapy to lift it to patency.

My notes from the Crumley conversation see him underscoring what the other two also stressed: the familial aspect of Lutheran life. He was aware that sometimes this occurs to the neglect of the single adults who make up one-third of mature Lutheranism—"but remember, singles are also part of families." He surmised, with Preus, that Lutherans would tilt toward *in vitro* fertilization as the techniques became more reliable and secure. Why? Because Lutheran tradition makes so much of the familial context that it wants to understand the impulse of couples to have children even when there are natural barriers against it. But families are not to be iso-lated: they must be clustered, collegial, congregating, if there is to be true support for health or in times of health crises.

For President Crumley as for the others, the Lutheran stress on the "priesthood of all believers" in respect to well-being meant less about de-mocracy in the church or lay autonomy and more about equal access to God. The congregants are all priests as intercessors. When Pope John Paul II said of his would-be assassin, "I will pray for you," that, smiled Crumley, "made him sound very Lutheran." "I will pray for you" is not meant to be a routine sound in the congregation but one part of the connection of care that also implies certain generosities, physical acts, and deep empathy as an instrument of support.

I left Keystone with a sense that the apparently elusive Lutheran tradi-tion, something about which the theologians in the main had not gotten around to applying to "well-being," *did* have subtle definitions. The out-lines are not clear, but there are what I call "zones" in which one is most aware of its palpability. A Studs Terkel interviewee once spoke of the "feel-ing tone" of a group or a way of life. Lutheranism proudly asserts its creeds, doggedly affirms dogma, rather prosaically lives its congregational life, and is all too apathetic about changing a world in which there need not be so much suffering. Yet in the midst of its yeses, noes, and maybes, its pluses and minuses, there does exist the glowing core, the center of coherence and a consequent "feeling tone." From it can come new contributions to the larger Christian search for well-being even as people in the tradition continue to learn from others, be they fellow Christian or not, who, under a provident God, promote human care and cure.

Notes

Chapter 1/Traditions and the Lutheran Tradition

1. Einar Billing, *Our Calling*, trans. Conrad Bergendoff (Rock Island, Ill.: Augustana Book Concern, 1947), pp. 7–11.
2. Leo Rosten, ed., *Religions in America* (New York: Simon and Schuster, 1975), pp. 160, 165.
3. Billing, p. 35.
4. W.H. Auden, "Luther," in *The Christian Century Reader*, ed. Harold E. Fey and Margaret Frakes (New York: Association Press, 1962), p. 433.
5. *The Book of Concord*, trans. and ed. Theodore G. Tappert (Philadelphia: Muhlenberg, 1959).
6. Philip Watson, *Let God Be God* (London: Epworth, 1947).
7. George Forell, *Faith Active in Love* (New York: The American Press, 1954).
8. Suzanne K. Langer, *Philosophy in a New Key* (New York: New American Library, 1952), pp. 39, 41.
9. Ortega, quoted in Harold C. Roley, *José Ortega y Gasset: Philosopher of European Unity* (University, Ala.: University of Alabama Press, 1971), p. 49.
10. *The Book of Concord*, pp. 411–13.
11. Pelikan, cited in A.R. Peacocke, *Creation and the World of Science* (Oxford: Clarendon Press, 1979), pp. 78–79.
12. *The Book of Concord*, pp. 412–13.
13. Heinrich Bornkamm, *Luther's World of Thought*, trans. Martin H. Bertram (St. Louis: Concordia, 1958), pp. 179–94.
14. Heinrich Bornkamm, *The Heart of Reformation Faith: The Fundamental Axioms of Evangelical Belief*, trans. John W. Doberstein (New York: Harper and Row, 1965), p. 110.
15. Werner Elert, *The Structure of Lutheranism*, trans. Walter A. Hansen (St. Louis: Concordia, 1962), pp. 407, 417.
16. Edmund Schlink, *Theology of the Lutheran Confessions*, trans. Paul F. Koehneke and Herbert J.A. Bouman (Philadelphia: Muhlenberg, 1961), pp. 38–40, 45.
17. Elert, pp. 452–562.
18. Quoted in A.R. Peacocke, p. 308.
19. Quoted in A.R. Peacocke, p. 297.
20. Quoted in Schlink, p. 59.

Chapter 2/Illness and Madness: The Issue of a Divine Role

1. Warren T. Reich, ed., *Encyclopedia of Bioethics*, 4 vols. (New York: Macmillan, 1978): 2:579–80.
2. Ibid., p. 582.
3. Ibid., p. 586.
4. Ibid., pp. 599–605.
5. Richard J. Jensen, *The Winning of the Midwest: Social and Political Conflict, 1888–*

1896 (Chicago: University of Chicago Press, 1971), pp. 83–84.

6. Oscar E. Feucht, et al., eds., *Sex and the Church: A Sociological, Historical, and Theological Investigation of Sex Attitudes* (St. Louis: Concordia, 1961), p. 85.

7. Claire Chambers, *The Siecus Circle: A Humanist Revolution* (Belmont: Western Islands, 1977), pp. 209–14.

8. Aarne Siirala, *The Voice of Illness* (Philadelphia: Fortress, 1964), pp. 30–133.

9. W.H. Auden, "Luther," in *The Christian Century Reader*, ed. Harold E. Fey and Margaret Frakes (New York: Association Press, 1962), p. 433.

Chapter 3/Suffering: The Theology of the Cross

1. Joseph H. Fichter, *Religion and Pain: The Spiritual Dimensions of Health Care* (New York: Crossroad, 1981), pp. 18–61.

2. Helmut Thielicke, *Death and Life*, trans. Edward H. Schroeder (Philadelphia: Fortress, 1970), p. 15.

3. Heinrich Bornkamm, *The Heart of Reformation Faith: The Fundamental Axioms of Evangelical Belief*, trans. John W. Doberstein (New York: Harper and Row, 1965), p. 115.

4. Dorothee Soelle, *Suffering* (Philadelphia: Fortress, 1975), pp. 21–30.

5. Harold Ditmanson, in an unpublished paper delivered at Keystone, Colorado, before a conference of Lutheran bishops, July 1982.

6. Quoted in Leonard Pinomaa, *Faith Victorious: An Introduction to Luther's Theology*, trans. by Walter J. Kukkonen (Philadelphia: Fortress, 1963), p. 1.

7. Walther von Loewenich, *Luther's Theology of the Cross*, trans. Herbert J.A. Bouman (Minneapolis: Augsburg, 1976), pp. 13ff, 119–23.

8. André Dumas, *Dietrich Bonhoeffer, Theologian of Reality* (New York: Macmillan,1971), pp. 203–7.

9. Jürgen Moltmann, *The Crucified God: The Cross of Christ as the Foundation and Criticism of Christian Theology*, trans. R.A. Wilson and John Bowden (New York: Harper and Row, 1974), pp. 233–34.

10. From the Weimar edition of Luther's works quoted in Werner Elert, *The Structure of Lutheranism*, trans. Walter A. Hansen (St. Louis: Concordia, 1962), pp. 467–68.

Chapter 4/Caring: Institutions, Roles, Practices

1. H. Richard Niebuhr, *Christ and Culture* (New York: Harper and Row, 1951).

2. John T. McNeill, *A History of the Cure of Souls* (New York: Harper and Row, 1951), pp. 163–71.

3. Theodore G. Tappert, ed., *Luther: Letters of Spiritual Counsel* (Philadelphia: Westminster,1955), pp. 13–17.

4. Milo L. Brekke, Merton P. Strommen, and Dorothy L. Williams, *Ten Faces of Ministry* (Minneapolis: Augsburg, 1979), pp. 62–65, 152–54.

5. John H.C. Fritz, *Pastoral Theology: A Handbook of Scriptural Principles Written Especially for Pastors of the Lutheran Church* (St. Louis: Concordia, 1932), pp. 123–24, 197.

6. G.H. Gerberding, *The Lutheran Pastor* (Philadelphia: Lutheran Publication Society, 1902), pp. 419–20, 432.

7. Granger Westberg, *Nurse, Pastor and Patient* (Rock Island, Ill.: Augustana Book Concern, 1955).

8. Wayne E. Oates, *Protestant Pastoral Counseling* (Philadelphia: Westminster, 1962), pp. 30–31.

9. Richard W. Solberg, *As Between Brothers: The Story of Lutheran Response to World Need* (Minneapolis: Augsburg, 1957), p. 56.

10. Cyril Eastwood, *The Priesthood of All Believers* (London: The Epworth Press, 1960), pp. 2–12, 61.

11. *Lutheran Health and Welfare Directory* (New York: Division of Welfare Services, Lutheran Council in the U.S.A., 1967).

12. William O. Shanahan, *German Protestants Face the Social Question* (Notre Dame: University of Notre Dame Press, 1954), pp. 3, 58–86.

Chapter 5/Healing: The Acts of Healing, the Arts of Prayer

1. Wade H. Boggs, Jr., *Faith, Healing and the Christian Faith* (Richmond: John Knox Press, 1956), p. 52.
2. Carl J. Scherzer, *The Church and Healing* (Philadelphia: Westminster, 1950), p. 68.
3. Larry Christenson, *The Charismatic Renewal Among Lutherans* (Minneapolis: Bethany Fellowship, 1976), pp. 94–112.
4. *Anointing and Healing* (Philadelphia: The United Lutheran Church Board of Publication, 1962), pp. 17–30, passim.
5. Peder Olsen, *Healing Through Prayer*, trans. John Jensen (Minneapolis: Augsburg, 1962), pp. 18–33.
6. *Health and Healing: The Report of the Makumira Consultation on the Healing Ministry of the Church* (Arusha: Medical Board of the Evangelical Lutheran Church in Tanzania, 1967), pp. 33–43.

Chapter 6/Morality, Ethics, and Justice: Being Good and Being Well

1. Warren T. Reich, ed., *The Encyclopedia of Bioethics*, 4 vols. (New York: Macmillan, 1978):1:400–407.
2. Richard F. Tomasson, *Iceland: The First New Society* (Minneapolis: University of Minnesota Press, 1980), pp. 84–199.
3. Lawrence K. Kersten, *The Lutheran Ethic: The Impact of Religion on Laymen and Clergy* (Detroit: Wayne State University Press, 1970), pp. 11–135.
4. Taken from *Faith and Ferment*, to be published by the Institute for Cultural and Ecumenical Research, Collegeville, Minnesota, pp. 6–7.
5. "Death and Dying," statement adopted by the 1982 convention of the Lutheran Church in America.
6. "Biomedical Ethics: Theological Perspectives," a study document produced in connection with the Lutheran Church in America project on biomedical ethics, 1980–1982, and available from the Lutheran Church in America, 231 Madison Avenue, New York, NY, 10016.
7. Ralph E. Peterson, *A Study of the Healing Church and Its Ministry* (New York: Lutheran Church in America, 1982), pp. 22–26.

Chapter 7/Sexuality, Family Life, and Generativity

1. F.V.N. Painter, *Luther on Education* (St. Louis: Concordia, 1928), pp. 113–14.
2. Martin Luther, *Predigt vom ehelichen Leben*, in *Luthers Werke*, vol. 3, Erlangen ed., p. 541, quoted in Paul Hansen et al., *Engagement and Marriage: A Sociological, Historical, and Theological Investigation of Engagement and Marriage* (St. Louis: Concordia, 1959), p. 67.
3. Derrick Sherwin Bailey, *Sexual Relations in Christian Thought* (New York: Harper and Brothers, 1959), p. 174.
4. Martin Luther, *Weimar Ausgabe, Briefe*, vol. 9, no. 3503; vol. 8, nos. 3423 and following (pp. 638–43); vol. 4, no. 1046; vol. 6, no. 1861, quoted in Hansen, *Engagement and Marriage*.
5. Oscar E. Feucht, et. al., eds, *Sex and the Church: A Sociological, Historical, and Theological Investigation of Sex Attitudes* (St. Louis: Concordia, 1961), p. 85.
6. Martin Luther, *Weimar Ausgabe*, vol. 40, p. 92; vol. 51, p. 52, quoted in William Lazareth, *Luther and the Christian Home* (Philadelphia: Muhlenberg, 1960), pp. 6, 32, 173.
7. All quotes from Hansen, pp. 5–114.
8. Harold E. Letts, ed., *Life in Community* (Philadelphia: Muhlenberg, 1957), p. 163.
9. Hansen, pp. 67, 95, 166–68.
10. Walter A. Maier, *For Better Not for Worse* (St. Louis: Concordia, 1939), pp. 410–11.
11. C.M. Zorn, quoted in Feucht, pp. 131–32.
12. William E. Hulme, *God, Sex and Youth* (Englewood Cliffs: Prentice-Hall, 1959), pp. 76, 77.
13. See Feucht, p. 79.
14. Quoted in Lazareth, pp. 185, 186, 193–94.

Chapter 8/The Passages of Life, the Phases of Faith

1. Quoted in Huston Smith, *Condemned to Meaning* (New York: Harper and Row, 1965), p. 14.

2. Victor Turner, *The Ritual Process: Structure and Anti-Structure* (Ithaca: Cornell University Press, 1969), pp. 166, 168.

3. George H. Williams, "Religious Residues and Presuppositions in the American Debate on Abortion," *Theological Studies* 31 (1970): 14, 41.

4. *Abortion: A Series of Statements of the American Lutheran Church, 1974, 1976, and 1980*; available from the American Lutheran Church, 422 S. Fifth Street, Minneapolis, Minn. 55415.

5. See "A Report of the Commission on Theology and Church Relations" in Victor B. Ficker and Herbert S. Graves, *The Revolution in Religion* (Columbus: Charles E. Merrill, 1973), pp. 139ff.

6. Ralph E. Peterson, *A Study of the Healing Church and Its Ministry* (New York: Lutheran Church in America, 1982), p. 14.

7. *The Book of Concord*, trans. and ed. Theodore G. Tappert (Philadelphia: Muhlenberg, 1959), pp. 442–45.

8. Gerald Strauss, *Luther's House of Learning: Indoctrination of the Young in the German Reformation* (Baltimore: Johns Hopkins Univ. Press, 1978), pp. 87–101.

9. Frank W. Klos, *Confirmation and First Communion* (Minneapolis: Augsburg, 1968), pp.47–55.

10. Peterson, p. 14.

11. *The Book of Concord*, p. 454.

Chapter 9/The Completion of Being, the Meaning of Dying

1. Philip Aries, *The Hour of Our Death* (New York: Knopf, 1981).

2. Ernest Becker, *The Denial of Death* (New York: Free Press, 1973).

3. Elisabeth Kübler-Ross, *On Death and Dying* (New York: Macmillan, 1971).

4. Dietrich Bonhoeffer, *The Communion of Saints: A Dogmatic Inquiry into the Sociology of the Church*, trans. R. Gregor Smith (New York: Harper and Row, 1963).

5. Heinrich Bornkamm, *Luther's World of Thought*, trans. Martin H. Bertram (St. Louis: Concordia, 1958), p. 115.

6. Helmut Thielicke, *Death and Life*, trans. Edward H. Schroeder (Philadelphia: Fortress, 1970), pp. 16, 144, 182, 147–59.

7. Heinrich Bornkamm, *The Heart of Reformation Faith: The Fundamental Axioms of Evangelical Belief*, trans. John W. Doberstein (New York: Harper and Row, 1965), pp. 117–30.